C
IMMUN

An Illustrated Outline

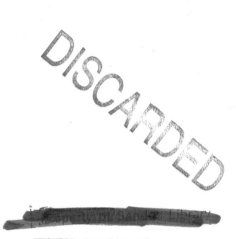

CLINICAL IMMUNOLOGY

An Illustrated Outline

Jonathan Brostoff

MA, DM (Oxon), DSc, FRCP, FRCPath.
Reader in Clinical Immunology
University College London
Medical School

David K. Male

MA, PhD
Senior Lecturer in Neuroimmunology
Department of Neuropathology
Institute of Psychiatry
London

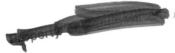

Project Manager	Mike Meakin
Illustrator	Lynda Payne
Production	Jane Tozer
Publisher	Harvey Shoolman

For full details of all Times Mirror International Publishers Limited titles, please write to Times
Mirror International Publishers Limited, Lynton House, 7–12 Tavistock Square, London WC1H
9LB, England.

A CIP catalogue record for this book is available from the British Library.

Library of Congress Cataloging-in-Publication Data (applied for)

How to use this book

This book serves two different functions. It can either be used as a dictionary of clinical immunology, or as a concise reference guide to the subject. Readers with some knowledge of immunolgy requiring a summary of particular aspects, should consult the contents page. The book is divided into eight sections each of which contains a number of topics set out on double page spreads.

To use this book as a dictionary, look up the word or abbreviation in the Index of Terms (pages 8 to 17). This gives a single page number where a definition of the word will be found – associated words and subjects are grouped on the same page. Page references to particular topics set out on several pages are indicated in **bold**; those in *italic* refer to figures.

Acknowledgements

We are most grateful to the individuals who have allowed us to use illustrations of clinical and histological material, which has previously appeared in the books *Immunology*, *Clinical Immunology* and *Immunology – An Illustrated Outline*. We thank Professor R.StC. Barnetson, Professor S. Challacombe, Professor A. Compston, Professor D.L. Easty, Dr G. Fahy, the late Professor H. Festenstein, Dr D. Gawkrodger, Professor M.F. Greaves, Dr A. Greening, Professor F. Hay, Dr D.P. Jewell, Dr T. Lund, Dr R. Mirakian, Dr A.J. Pinching, Dr M. Snaith, Professor M. Steward, Dr P. Sweny and Dr T. Hall, as well as our co-editors Glenis Scadding and Ivan Roitt.

A book of this kind cannot include everything of interest to immunologists, nor have we been able to cover every disease which has immune system involvement. Nevertheless, we have tried to cover all the key areas of basic immunology, relating this to the more commonly encountered clinical conditions. If readers consider that additional subjects should be included or deserve further detail, we would be pleased to hear from them.

Contents

Index of terms

A

ABO
  blood group antigens 27
  secretor status 27
Acquired immune deficiency
  syndrome (AIDS) **78**
Acute
  lymphoblastic
    leukaemias (ALL) 96
Addison's disease 40
Adenosine deaminase
  (ADA) deficiency *70*, 72
Adherence technique 122
Adjuvants 109
Adrenal autoimmunity 40
Adult
  respiratory distress syn-
    drome (ARDS) 91
  T cell leukaemia (ATL)
    97
AFCs (Antibody forming
  cells) 20
Affinity of antibodies 113
Agranulocytosis 95
AIHA (Autoimmune
  haemolytic anaemia) 60
AIDS **78**
  neuropathology 79
  -related complex (ARC)
    78
ALG (Anti-lymphocyte glob-
  ulin) 107
Allergic
  bronchopulmonary
    aspergillosis 91
  contact dermatitis 66
  ophthalmic disorders 54
Allorecognition 102
Alternative pathway defi-
  ciencies 76
Amoxycillin 48
Amyloidosis 45
Anaphylaxis *131*

Ankylosing spondylitis (AS)
  33
Anti
  -DNA antibodies 35
  -glomerular basement
    membrane antibody-
    mediated GN 43
  -lymphocyte antibodies
    107
  -lymphocyte globulin
    (ALG) 107
Antibodies 21
  affinity and avidity 113
  assays **114**
  cross-reactivity 113
  specificity 112
Antibody
  forming cells (AFCs) 20
  titre 113
Antigen
  assays **114**
  presenting cells (APCs)
    21
Antigenic variation 110
Antigens, nuclear,
  extractable 35
Antiglobulin (Coombs) test
  27
Antimitochondrial antibodies
  53
Antineutrophil cytoplasmic
  antibody (ANCA) 44
APCs (Antigen presenting
  cells) 21
ARC (AIDS-related com-
  plex) 78
ARDS (Adult respiratory distress syndrome) 91
Arthritis, reactive 33
AS (Ankylosing spondylitis)
  33
Ascaris infestation 58
Aspergillus fumigatus 59

13

Introduction   1

The immune system has evolved to protect individuals from infectious micro-organisms. This process of protection requires lymphocytes to recognize the infectious agent and then mount an appropriate immune response, which can either eliminate the pathogen or minimize the damage it causes. During the initial recognition phase the immune system must distinguish molecules expressed by the pathogen (antigens) from those expressed by the host. In the second, effector phase of the immune response, the appropriate response will depend on the type of infection and its localization. The immune system must be capable of dealing with intracellular pathogens such as viruses, some bacteria and protozoal parasites: it must also handle extracellular pathogens and their toxins, including many bacteria, multicellular parasites and free virus. In general, T lymphocytes are responsible for the recognition of antigens originating from within cells of the body, while antibodies (produced by B lymphocytes), in association with phagocytic cells and the complement system, deal with extracellular pathogens and antigens. The system of immune recognition and response can break down in many ways, and can lead to the problems encountered by clinical immunologists.

Autoimmunity and autoimmune disease. The immune system generates antibodies and T cell receptors (TCRs), which can recognize a very wide variety of antigens, including host molecules. These are generated before encounter with the antigen. However, lymphocytes do not usually react against the individual's own tissues – a condition referred to as autoimmunity. This is partly due to the process of T cell education during thymic development, and partly to a series of checks and controls on autoimmune reactions. Where these controls break down, immune effector mechanisms may be brought to bear, and autoimmune disease results.

Immunodeficiency occurs when the immune system is unable to make an adequate immune response and so fails to control a pathogen. Primary immunodeficiencies may be caused by genetic abnormality in any of the arms of the immune system. Secondary deficiencies are due to external factors, such as viruses, toxins or malnutrition.

Hypersensitivity occurs when the damage produced by an immune response to the host tissue is greater than that caused by the inducing pathogen or antigen. The line dividing an appropriate immune response from hypersensitivity depends on the pathogen and the tissue involved. For example: 1) an innocuous antigen such as pollen may induce a strong inflammatory reaction in the nasal mucosa or lung (see Fig. 1.1); and 2) some viruses that infect neurones do not kill the neurones themselves, but they may stimulate the immune system to destroy the infected cell.

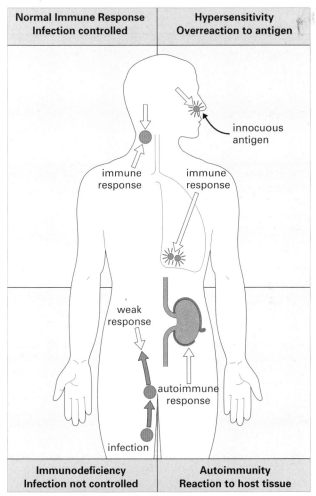

Fig. 1.1 Normal and pathogenic immune responses.

ELEMENTS OF THE IMMUNE SYSTEM

CD system Leucocytes are distinguished according to the groups of molecules that they express on their surfaces. Most molecules have been classified into the 'CD' system, which defines more than 130 cell surface molecules distinguishable by monoclonal antibodies. These molecules may be lineage specific or shared between different cell types. Some appear only at particular stages of cell development, and others only on activated cells. Figure 1.2 lists the most useful markers of particular cells.

T cells are responsible for recognizing antigens presented by other cells of the body. Cytotoxic T cells (Tc) are mostly CD8$^+$, and recognize cells infected with virus, which they can then kill. Helper T cells (TH) are CD4$^+$ and recognize antigens that have been taken up by antigen-presenting cells and which express antigen fragments on the cell surface. Helper T cells interact directly with other cells by releasing cytokines to control the development of immune responses. There are two main sets of T helper cells:1) TH1 cells activate macrophages, causing them to destroy material they have taken up; 2) TH2 cells help B cells to make antibody. The balance of activity between the different TH sets determines the type of immune response that will develop.

Cytokines are soluble proteins released by cells (primarily activated T cells), which act as signals between cells of the immune system and may also act on other cells of the body. There are four major groups of cytokines: 1) the interleukins (IL-1 to IL-12); 2) the interferons (IFN-α, IFN-β and IFN-γ); 3) the colony stimulating factors (CSFs); and 4) the tumour necrosis factors (TNF-α and TNF-β, also called lymphotoxin).

Mononuclear phagocytes/monocytes/macrophages Cells of this lineage are long-lived, and distributed throughout the body. They express receptors for antibody and activated complement components, which they use to take up immune complexes. Blood monocytes differentiate into macrophages in tissues, and any cell of this lineage can act as an antigen presenting cell.

B cells/antibody forming cells (AFCs)/plasma cells are the group of lymphocytes that produce antibody. B cells differentiate into antibody forming cells, which are recognized histologically as plasma cells. Each clone of B cells uses a distinct surface antibody to recognize antigen, and will ultimately secrete antibody of this specificity.

Antibodies/immunoglobulins (Igs) are produced by B cells and bind specifically to antigenic determinants (epitopes) on antigens. There are five main classes of antibody: 1) IgG; 2) IgA; 3) IgM; 4) IgD; and 5) IgE. IgG is the main serum antibody; it can directly neutralize some antigens and it facilitates uptake of others by phagocytes carrying antibody receptors (Fc receptors). IgA is the main secreted antibody.

Antigen presenting cells (APCs) are a functionally defined group of cells which can present antigen to $CD4^+$ T cells. They include dendritic cells, macrophages and B cells, but other cell types may act as antigen presenting cells during disease.

Complement system is a group of serum molecules and cell surface receptors involved in the control of inflammation. The main functions are: 1) opsonization of antigen/antibody complexes, for endocytosis by phagocytes; 2) lysis of plasma membranes of cells and some pathogens sensitized by antibody; 3) attraction of macrophages and neutrophils to sites of inflammation; 4) activation of mast cells and basophils to release mediators controlling blood flow, capillary permeability and leucocyte accumulation.

Natural killer (NK) cells/null cells/large granular lymphocytes (LGLs) are lymphocytes lacking a T or B cell phenotype, but with some non-specific anti-viral or anti-tumour activity.

Cell type	Marker	Function
T cells	CD2	adhesion & non-specific activation
	CD3	part of T cell antigen receptor (TCR)
TH subsets	mostly CD4	MHC class II receptor
TC subset	mostly CD8	MHC class I receptor
B cells	CD19, CD20	differentiation markers
	surface Ig	antigen receptor
mononuclear	CD64	antibody receptor (FcγR1)
phagocytes	CD11b	complement receptor (CR3)
activated T cells	CD25	interleukin-2 receptor (IL–2R)
B cells &	CD71	transferrin receptor
macrophages		

Fig. 1.2 **Principle CD markers.**

THE MAJOR HISTOCOMPATIBILITY COMPLEX (MHC)

The MHC is a set of genes located on chromosome 6 in man. This region contains at least 80 genes, which may be divided into four main groups – classes I to IV. These genes were first identified, because of their role in graft rejection – it was found that individuals who have identical sets of MHC genes would usually accept grafts from each other, whereas individuals with different loci would not. It is now known that the class I and class II genes encode molecules that are involved in communication between cells of the body and T lymphocytes.

Human leucocyte antigen (HLA) 'Locus' is the name given to the MHC in man. It is so called because the class I and class II molecules were first identified on the surface of leucocytes.

MHC class I genes (HLA-A, HLA-B and HLA-C) encode molecules expressed on the surface of all nucleated cells. Class I molecules bind to peptides of other molecules produced within the cell and transport them to the cell surface where the complex of MHC class I and peptide may be recognized by CD8$^+$ cytotoxic T cells. This allows the T cells to recognize and kill any cell of the body productively infected with virus.

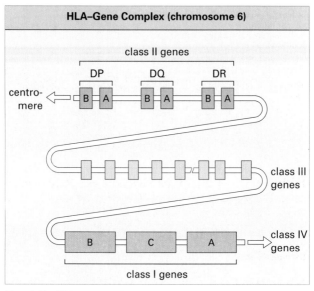

Fig. 1.3 The HLA gene complex (chromosome 6).

MHC class II genes (HLA-DP, HLA-DQ and HLA-DR) encode molecules expressed on the surface of a restricted group of cells, functionally defined as antigen presenting cells (APCs). Class II molecules bind to peptides of molecules that the APC has internalized. The complex of MHC class II and peptide is then expressed at the cell surface where it can be recognized by CD4$^+$ T cells. This process of antigen presentation and T cell stimulation initiates immune responses and partly determines the type of response which will occur.

MHC class III genes encode a large number of diverse proteins, including some complement components (C2, C4 and factor B), the cytokines tumour necrosis factor (TNF) and lymphotoxin (LT), a number of enzymes, certain heat shock proteins, and transporter molecules involved in antigen processing.

MHC class IV genes are structurally similar to class I genes, but are mostly expressed during development.

MHC molecules This term usually refers specifically to the cell surface molecules (HLA antigens) encoded by the class I and class II MHC gene loci. Class I molecules have one chain (α) encoded within the MHC which associates with a polypeptide (β_2-microglobulin) encoded outside the MHC. The class II loci – DP, DQ and DR – have two MHC-encoded chains (α and β). 'A' genes encode α chains and 'B' genes β chains. The number of B genes in the DR locus varies with different haplotypes.

Polymorphism refers to variation between individuals of a species at a particular gene locus. The MHC class I and II loci are extremely polymorphic, with at least 24 structural variants of HLA-A, 50 of HLA-B and 11 of HLA-C. The HLA-DR locus is the most polymorphic class II locus with at least 20 variants (see Appendix IV). Variation at the DNA level is even greater than the polymorphism at the protein level.

Haplotype refers to a set of genes on a single (haploid) chromosome. The great majority of individuals inherit a different MHC haplotype from each parent. As MHC genes are codominately expressed, this means that cells may produce up to six different MHC class I molecules. Expression of class II molecules on APCs is similarly diverse.

HLA AND DISEASE

Disease association It has been observed that different HLA genes are associated with increased susceptibility to, or protection from, particular diseases. A disease association occurs when a particular MHC haplotype is over-represented in an affected population, by comparison with ethnically matched controls. Most diseases involving immune reactions show some disease associations, but they are particularly notable in the various autoimmune conditions.

Relative risk is a measure of the risk of an individual with a particular haplotype contracting a specific disease. A relative risk greater than 1 denotes greater suspectibility, while less than 1 indicates some protection. For example, individuals with HLA-B27 are 90 times more likely to contract ankylosing spondylitis than individuals lacking this class I gene.

HLA typing is used to determine an individual's HLA class I and II haplotypes. This is sometimes valuable as an aid to diagnosis, where a disease has a strong MHC association: it is essential in matching donors and recipients for transplantation. Currently the great majority of HLA typing is carried out using monoclonal antibodies specific for each HLA locus and haplotype, using the patient's lymphocytes. It is also possible to differentiate class II loci using 'mixed lymphocyte cultures' or 'primed lymphocyte typing'. In these assays, lymphocytes that lack a particular class II haplotype are stimulated to divide in the presence of stimulating cells which do express it.

The polypeptides of the different HLA haplotypes vary in their amino acid sequences, but there is additional variability in the DNA, detectable by molecular biological techniques. This has lead to a nomenclature system which indicates variation at both protein and DNA levels.

HLA haplotype nomenclature An individual MHC haplotype variant is indicated by its gene locus and a four-digit number. For example HLA-B*2702 is a variant of the class I HLA-B locus. The first two digits correspond to the closest serological specificity (B-27), and the second two indicate the variant number carrying that specificity.

Linkage is the term used to describe the way in which different genes on a single chromosome are linked together, and usually transmitted to offspring as a single block. For example, a single link-age group might consist of: HLA—DPw4—DQw3—DR9—B8—Cw11—A3—.

Linkage disequilibrium Over evolutionary time, the different MHC variants should become randomly associated with other variants by genetic recombination. Sometimes, however, particular variants are more frequently associated than chance predicts (e.g. HLA-A3 and -B7). This is called linkage disequilibrium, and may be due to a selective advantage in their association or because insufficient time has passed for them to distribute themselves randomly.

MHC expression and function. Class I molecules are expressed on all nucleated cells, where they present antigens from inside that cell to CD8$^+$ T cells. Class II molecules are constitutively expressed on a small group of antigen presenting cells, including dendritic cells, B cells and some macrophages. They may also be induced on a variety of other cell types during immune reactions *in vivo*, or by interferon-γ. They present partly degraded antigens which the cell has internalized, to CD4$^+$ T cells.

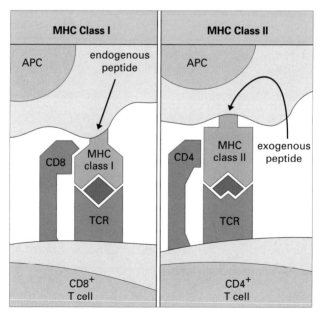

Fig. 1.4 **Functions of MHC molecules.**

BLOOD GROUPS

Blood groups are sets of allelically variable molecules expressed on the surface of erythrocytes, and sometimes on other cells. They may be protein or carbohydrate, but they have the ability to induce specific antibodies when transfused into individuals lacking that variant. These antibodies can then haemolyse the transfused cells. Autoantibodies to red cells, platelets and leucocytes may also occur, but these are usually directed to different antigens to those which induce alloantibodies.

Haemolysis Antibodies to red cells, particularly IgM, IgG1 and IgG3, can cause intravascular haemolysis by activating the complement system. IgG antibodies may also sensitize red cells for elimination by splenic macrophages – extravascular haemolysis.

System	Gene Loci	Phenotype frequencies (caucasoids)		Antibodies
ABO	1	A B AB O	42% 8% 3% 47%	naturally occurring IgM
Rhesus	3 linked major antigen = Rh–D	$Rh–D^+$ $Rh–D^-$	85% 15%	induced IgG
Kell	1	K k	9% 91%	induced, usually IgG
Duffy	1	Fy^aFy^b Fy^a Fy^b Fy	46% 20% 34% 0.1%	induced IgG
Kidd	1	Jk^a Jk^b	80% 19%	induced IgG
MNS P Lutheran	antigens antigens antigens	M or N P or p Lu^a or Lu^b		These systems are weakly immunogenic

Fig. 1.5 Human blood group systems.

ABO blood group antigens are widely distributed throughout the body, and act as histocompatibility antigens. They are determined by the A, B and O alleles on chromosome 9, which are codominately expressed – individuals are AB, A, B or O. The antigens themselves are complex carbohydrates synthesized by enzymes encoded at the ABO locus. This group is particularly important as individuals lacking an allelic variant spontaneously develop antibodies to that antigen, without exposure to incompatible blood or tissue.

ABO secretor status About 80% of individuals have the gene 'Se' and produce soluble forms of the ABO antigens.

Rhesus (Rh) blood group is determined by a gene complex giving rise to combinations of C or c, D or d and E or e. The major antigen is Rhesus-D, which induces (mostly) IgG antibodies in sensitized individuals. It is the most common system implicated in haemolytic disease of the newborn.

Kell blood group is encoded by a single locus with allotypes K and k, the K antigen being of greater immunogenicity. This group is the second most common in haemolytic disease of the newborn.

Antiglobulin (Coombs) test is widely used to identify autoantibodies or transfusion-induced antibodies to red cells, which cause haemagglutination. Some blood-group-specific antibodies directly agglutinate red cells, but those that do not are still detectable by adding anti-immunoglobulin to crosslink the Ig-sensitized red cells.

Platelet antigens Several allelically variable sets of platelet specific antibodies have been identified. Antibodies to these antigens may be induced by repeated transfusion and these may be associated with post transfusion purpura. Neonatal thrombocytopenia can occur in children of sensitized mothers.

Neutrophil (leucocyte) antigens Several sets of neutrophil-specific antigens have been identified, in addition to HLA molecules, which are distributed on other cell types. Antibodies may be induced by transfusion or occur as idiopathic autoantibodies or in association with other conditions, including systemic lupus erythematosus, Felty's syndrome and autoimmune haemolytic anaemias and thrombocytopenias.

Autoimmunity   2

Autoimmunity describes the reactions of autoreactive T cells or autoantibodies with self molecules. These may recruit effector systems to produce autoimmune diseases. Several potential mechanisms may lead to autoimmunity: 1.Cross-reaction with microbial antigens. Some micro-organisms have epitopes which also occur on self molecules. An immune reaction against such antigens may induce T cells reacting with the pathogen to help B cells producing autoantibodies. This occurs for example in rheumatic fever. 2.Polyclonal activation. Some infections such as malaria or EB virus can polyclonally activate B cells. The antibodies induced include a number of self molecules. 3.Immune disregulation may be due to a variety of causes acting in combination. Factors cited include aberrant processing and presentation of self molecules, due to infection or enhanced MHC inducibility, low levels of inhibitory cytokines (e.g. TGFβ) or protracted responses and sensitivity to activating cytokines (e.g. IL-2). A failure of central T cell self-tolerance may occur in diseases such as myasthenia gravis.

Autoimmune diseases occur as a spectrum. At one end the disease is limited to one organ of the body (e.g. Hashimoto's thyoiditis); at the other pole, antibodies are directed against widely distributed antigens, and the disease process is also widely disseminated. This is typified by systemic lupus erythematosus (SLE). Thus autoimmunity is classified into organ-specific and non-organ-specific diseases. Overlap occurs at each end of the spectrum. For example, patients with pernicious anaemia and gastric autoimmunity often have thyroid autoantibodies. Similarly, there is a cluster of diseases at the non-organ-specific end, including rheumatoid arthritis and SLE. Overlap between diseases at either end of the spectrum is rare.

Autoantibodies increase with age in the community, but this is not usually associated with disease. Autoantibodies may be primary, directly producing disease (e.g. in Goodpasture's syndrome) or may develop secondarily following tissue damage and release of self antigens where the response is often transient. Even when autoantibodies are not pathogenic they may provide a useful marker for diagnosis. A wide variety of autoantibody tests are carried out in clinical immunology laboratories and may predict disease, as well as signify its presence.

Aetiology of autoimmunity Genetic factors are important in autoimmune disease, but environmental factors also clearly play a part. This is demonstrated in studies of identical twins where the concordance rate in the various autoimmune diseases rarely exceeds 60%. Particular MHC haplotypes frequently contribute towards disease susceptibility, particularly the haplotypes HLA-A1, -B8 and -DR3. Infectious agents can induce autoimmunity by cross reaction, polyclonal activation or the induction of tissue damage and altered antigen presentation, as noted above.

Pathogenesis of autoimmune diseases can sometimes be related to the level of autoantibodies. For example in neonatal thyrotoxicosis, IgG thyroid-stimulating autoantibodies cross the placenta and induce thyrotoxicosis in the child. For many diseases however, cell-mediated immune reactions are at least as important, as disease cannot be induced by antibodies alone. The mechanisms cited include cytotoxic T cells, acting directly, or by releasing toxic cytokines, or by activating macrophages to release enzymes, reactive oxygen intermediates (ROIs), etc.

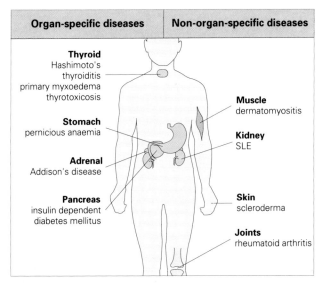

Fig. 2.1 Types of autoimmunity: organ-specific and non-organ-specific.
Although the non-organ-specific diseases produce symptoms in different organs, particular organs are more markedly affected by particular diseases.

Rheumatoid Diseases

Rheumatoid arthritis (RA)

Clinical features are those of an inflammatory disease of the synovium which results in erosion, destruction and deformity of the joints. The female to male ratio is 3:1 and the prevalence in the population is 1–3%. The most important feature of the disease is joint erosion which leads to deformity and disability.

Extra-articular disease affects a third of the patients and consists of: 1) fibrosing alveolitis with pulmonary interstitial inflammation and oedema; 2) vasculitis affecting the skin, nerves and eyes; 3) granuloma formation with focal necrosis with cell infiltration. The prognosis is always worse when there is extra-articular disease. Nodules and vasculitis indicate severe joint disease.

Felty's syndrome shows prominent vasculitis with lymphoid hyperplasia, enlarged liver/spleen and leucopenia in patients with RA.

Pathology of the joint shows early proliferation of the lining cells of the synovium which can result in villous hypertrophy with cell infiltration and aggregation into lymphoid follicles where the majority of the cells are T cells. Finger-like processes of the synovial tissue extend into the cartilage as pannus leading to erosion of the cartilage and bone (Figures 2.2 and 2.3).

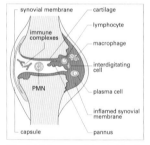

Fig. 2.2 Rheumatoid arthritis. An inflammatory infiltrate is found in the synovial membrane which hypertrophies, covering and eventually eroding the synovial cartilage and bone. Immune complexes and polymorphonuclear leucocytes are detectable in the joint space.

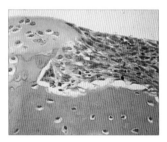

Fig. 2.3 Histology of pannus, seen as a layer of lymphocytes, macrophages and plasma cells overlying and eroding the cartilage. Note the tissue destruction at the pannus margin. The layer below the cartilage is bone. (H & E stain.)

Cytokines are secreted in the rheumatoid synovium; GM-CSF and TNF-α, which stimulate the macrophages to secrete further TNF-α, IL-1 and IL-6. There is little IFN-γ or TNF-β despite the presence of mRNA. This might be the inhibitory effect of TGF, another cytokine.

Autoantibodies. The most important autoantibodies are the rheumatoid factors (RF), which react with the patient's own immunoglobulin. The antigenic site spans the CH2 and CH3 domains of the Fc fragment. They are typically IgM anti-IgG, but can be of other classes. Antinuclear autoantibodies (ANA) are present in half the patients but are of the IgM class and of low titre. C-reactive protein can be raised and this can distinguish active RA from systemic lupus erythematosus (SLE), where the level is usually normal.

Seronegative patients with RA fall into two groups: those with moderate disease, about 30% who do not have rheumatoid factors (RFs) – so-called seronegative – and the majority with more severe disease, who have RFs and therefore have seropositive RA. The presence of RF is not diagnostic of RA but does have value in prognosis.

Immune complexes in the joint and blood consist of IgG, IgM and complement, suggesting that IgG is the 'antigen'. Where the disease is limited to the joint, immune complexes are mainly in the joint fluid and tend to be lacking in the blood. With systemic disease they are present in both compartments. Circulating immune complexes can cause vasculitis and can lead to symptoms similar to SLE. Unlike SLE, immune complex nephritis is rare in RA.

Glycosylation of IgG may be relevant to RA. The immunoglobulin molecule (IgG) in patients with RA has less carbohydrate, lacking in galactose. In normal subjects, 14% of the IgG Fc sugar groups lack the terminal galactose, compared with 60% in RA. Abnormally glycosylated IgG is also found in patients with tuberculosis.

Diagnosis is based on clinical grounds with symmetrical polyarthritis and erosions seen on X-ray. The immunological test of the most value is that for RFs, which, if present in high titre, support the diagnosis. SLE would be indicated if antibodies to DNA were present; anti-Ro (SS-A) or anti-La (SS-B) would suggest Sjögren's syndrome. Tests for the presence of immune complexes are difficult to perform, lack reproducibility and are now rarely used for diagnosis.

Aetiology. Hormonal factors are important as RA is more common in women than in men, onset is usually after the menarche and before the menopause and the disease improves during pregnancy. Genetic factors are shown as the disease runs in families and there is an association with DR-4 and to a lesser extent with DR-1.

Infectious agents are thought to trigger RA in a genetically susceptible host. However isolation from the joints of any particular infectious agent has never been consistent. Cross reactivity of DR-4 with a surface antigen of *Proteus vulgaris* and the persistence of this organism in the urinary tract, especially of women, throws an interesting new light on a possible aetiology of the disease.

Diet and arthritis There is controversy as to the role of diet in RA. Rabbits and pigs fed on particular foods develop an arthritis similar to RA. There are two sorts of diet. One involves increasing poly-unsaturated fatty acids which favours the production of E3 prostaglandins and leukotrienes from eicosapentenoic acid. These fatty acids are less inflammatory than those of the E2 series produced from arachidonic acid metabolism.

Food intolerance Studies now show that elimination diets are useful in relieving symptoms in a proportion of patients with RA. Follow-up of patients on elimination diets suggest a significant long term effect. Identification of the culprit foods is difficult but worthwhile.

Drug treatment. First-line non-steroidal anti-inflammatory drugs (NSAIDs) such as aspirin and other prostaglandin synthetase inhibitors, indomethacin and ibuprofen. Second-line drugs such as gold salts (Myocrisine), D-penicillamine, sulphasalazine and chloroquine. Third-line drugs are steroids and cytotoxic drugs (prednisolone, azathioprine, cyclophosphamide and methotrexate). Recently, monoclonal antibodies against CD-4 have shown benefit in severe disease.

Juvenile chronic arthritis (JCA) (Still's disease)
By definition the onset is under the age of 16 years, and the duration has to be greater than 3 months. It can now be divided into four types.

Juvenile rheumatoid arthritis is the equivalent of adult RA, and is associated with DR4 and the presence of rheumatoid factor. There are joint erosions with destructive arthritis and it tends to be more severe than the adult disease. This group comprises 10% of chronic arthritis in children. Treatment is as for adults.

Pauciarticular JCA is seen in very young children and is associated with DR5 and DR8. The large joints tend to be affected. The patients are seronegative, although some have ANA which can be associated with iridocyclitis which can lead to blindness. This group comprises 50% of the JCA patients.

Polyarticular JCA affects mainly girls with small joints being involved. Those that present young have a better prognosis and represent 10% of this group.

Systemic JCA presents with fever, rash, lymphadenopathy, enlarged liver/spleen and pericarditis and comprises 15% of the group. There are no known serological markers and the disease can run a protracted course. Treatment is aggressive with steroids and cytotoxic drugs.

Seronegative spondyloarthropathies
The patients in this group do not have RF and the arthritis usually involves the spine. These conditions are more common in men and the onset is in the late teens or early twenties. The arthritis is strongly associated with HLA-B27.

Ankylosing spondylitis (AS) involves the spine and sacroiliac joints with ankylosis (fusion), which gives the X-ray appearance of bamboo spine. 95% of the patients are HLA-B27. Untreated cases may develop a fused and immobile vertebral column. A surface antigen on *Klebsiella pneumoniae* cross-reacts with HLA-B27. IgA and IgG anti-*Klebsiella* antibodies are also at higher titres in AS patients. A low carbohydrate diet results in a fall in anti-*Klebsiella* antibodies (and total IgA), a reduction in acute phase proteins and a significant clinical improvement. This is a good example of molecular mimicry.

Reactive arthritis appears to follow an infection and 60% of patients are HLA-B27 positive. The infections may be associated with organisms such as *Salmonella*, *Shigella* and *Yersinia*, or with *Chlamydia* in the cases of non-gonococcal genitourinary infections.

Reiter's syndrome applies to the triad of urethritis, arthritis and uveitis and complicates 1% of cases with non-specific urethritis and 2% of cases of dysentery; 75% of cases are HLA-B27 positive.

Inflammatory bowel disease such as ulcerative colitis, Crohn's disease and coeliac disease can all be associated with an arthritis similar to reactive arthritis. It may be due to absorption of bacterial components from a gut that has abnormal permeability due to the chronic inflammation. Treatment of the bowel disease often results in an improvement in the joint symptoms.

Psoriasis is associated with arthritis that may be similar to RA or reactive arthritis. Arthritis mutilans is a rare pattern of joint disease unique to psoriasis. The diagnosis may be missed either because the psoriasis escapes notice or because the joint disease precedes the skin condition. Treating the skin can improve the arthritis.

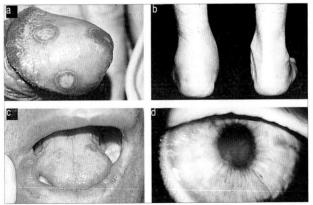

Fig. 2.4 Reiter's syndrome. Characterized by (a) urethritis and balanitis of the penis, (b) thickening of the Achilles tendon left, (c) mouth ulcers, and (d) inflammation of the iris (iritis).

SYSTEMIC LUPUS ERYTHEMATOSUS AND OTHER CONNECTIVE TISSUE DISORDERS

Systemic lupus erythematosus

Clinical features are those of a multisystem disease affecting many organs of the body. The typical patient is a young woman between 20 and 40 years old with a facial rash in the 'butterfly' area and arthralgia. There may be protein and red cells in the urine, and many other features of the disease such as anaemia, leucopenia, raised erythrocyte sedimentation rate (ESR) and elevated globulin levels. A summary of the clinical findings is shown in Figure 2.5.

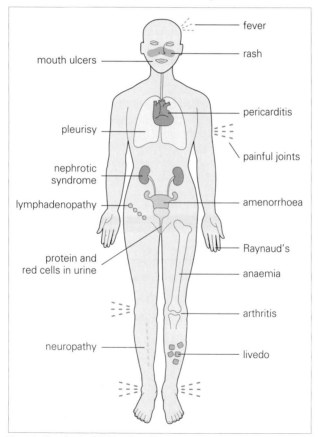

Fig. 2.5 The classical SLE patient. The patient often loses hair rapidly during active disease, sometimes with frank alopecia. Headaches are common and may be migrainous. Other symptoms are as indicated in the figure.

Diagnosis is made on clinical findings, and the detection of the classical antinuclear autoantibodies (ANA) in the serum. Over 95% of patients with SLE have ANA.

Anti-DNA antibodies are characteristic of SLE. The most specific form are against double-stranded DNA (dsDNA), measured using the double immunofluorescence on *Crithidia luciliae*. Antibodies against single-stranded DNA (ssDNA) are found in a number of diseases, including infections and other autoimmune conditions. Although DNA–anti-DNA complexes are found at sites of tissue inflammation, DNA itself has not been found in circulating immune complexes.

Extractable nuclear antigens also induce autoantibodies. These do not have the same specificity for the diagnosis of SLE as ANA but are useful in the diagnosis of overlap syndromes such as mixed connective tissue disease (MCTD). In this condition, antibodies to RNP are necessary for the diagnosis. Anti-Ro/La are present in Sjögren's syndrome and anti-Jo 1 in polymyositis.

Lupus 'band' test is seen on biopsy of uninvolved skin and shows complement and immunoglobulin deposition at the junction of the dermis and epidermis. It is not specific for SLE but is of diagnostic help.

Lupus anticoagulant syndrome

This syndrome consists of recurrent abortions, venous and arterial thromboses and thrombocytopenia. The lupus anticoagulant is an autoantibody directed against the Factor X clotting complex and causes a prolonged clotting time *in vitro* but thrombosis *in vivo*. There is overlap between the clinical presentation of this syndrome and that of the primary antiphospholipid antibody syndrome, which can occur together but do have separate antibodies.

HLA associations are with the haplotype HLA-A1, B8, DR3. The link with HLA-B27 and ankylosing spondylitis, and DR4 with the synovitis of rheumatoid arthritis are not seen in SLE.

Pathogenesis. The disease process is regarded as an immune complex disorder although the level of circulating complexes does not correlate well with either disease activity or clinical features.

Drug-induced lupus

A patient who is DR4-positive, a slow acetylator, is already hypertensive and who is receiving hydralazine may well develop drug-induced lupus. This condition often settles when the drug is withdrawn, although the ANA may remain. Other drugs such as procainamide, some antibiotics, anticonvulsants and penicillamine may rarely cause the same syndrome.

Treatment is aimed at reducing immune complex deposition and also providing symptomatic relief for the patient.

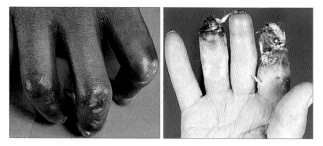

Fig. 2.6 (Left) **Scleroderma:** the skin on the hands is thickened and tethered; (right) **gangrene** due to obliterative vasculopathy.

Prognosis has improved considerably. The 5-year survival of all forms of SLE is now greater than 90% and is only slightly lower for patients with nephritis. Pregnancy is associated with a higher rate of stillbirth and spontaneous abortion but is not contraindicated in patients with SLE. Infection is the most common cause of death.

Scleroderma

The word 'scleroderma' describes thickening of the skin and its tethering to subcutaneous tissue. The syndrome **progressive systemic sclerosis** includes smooth muscle atrophy and fibrosis of internal organs. Renal involvement with accelerated hypertension is the complication most likely to be fatal. There are numerous subtypes, including CREST syndrome and clinical features depend on the organ(s) affected.

Pathology shows increased collagen deposition in the skin (Figure 2.6), subcutaneous tissues and internal organs. Microscopic changes around arterioles and capillaries show perivascular inflammation with cellular infiltrates leading to obliteration of the vessels or dilatation. All these changes can be found in the skin and internally.

Autoantibodies and in particular ANA, are found in 90% of patients, with the nucleolar pattern being characteristic. Antibody to soluble nuclear antigen, Scl-70 although specific for scleroderma is only found in 25% of patients. Anti-centromere antibody is associated with the sclerodactyly of the CREST syndrome.

Graft versus host disease

When delayed and chronic, this syndrome shows many similarities with scleroderma, but there are also features of Sjögren's syndrome, SLE and primary biliary cirrhosis.

Diagnosis of scleroderma is based on clinical findings. The results of autoantibodies are useful, skin and renal biopsy not being routinely necessary. Nail-fold capillary microscopy is a useful and simple clinical method of confirming the vascular abnormalities.

Treatment includes corticosteroids, colchicine, D-penicillamine and immunosuppression. Controlled trials have been few and inconclusive.

Sjögren's syndrome

The term originally described patients with arthritis and dry eyes and mouth. The arthritis is rheumatoid in type and the term sicca is used to denote the variable aspects of mucosal dryness. The syndrome can be divided into **primary Sjögren's**, i.e. the sicca syndrome; **secondary Sjögren's**, which includes SLE, primary biliary cirrhosis, polymyositis and SLE with the sicca syndrome; and **Sjögren's syndrome with rheumatoid arthritis**. Primary Sjögren's syndrome characteristically shows exocrine gland abnormality with dryness affecting eyes, mouth, lung and vagina. Systemic features are not marked, apart from fatigue and arthralgia. Some may show signs similar to SLE with Raynaud's phenomenon or vasculitis.

Autoantibodies. Anti-Ro and anti-La have also been described as anti-SS-A and anti-SS-B are present in some patients with Sjögren's syndrome. ANA are found in all types of Sjögren's patients and do not indicate a particular disease severity. Rheumatoid factors are present in 1% of Sjögren's patients but do not correlate with cartilage erosions as they do in rheumatoid arthritis.

Salivary gland pathology is specific and shows mononuclear and lymphocyte (CD4$^+$) infiltrates around the salivary ducts, with class II expression and EBV DNA. This suggests autoreactive lymphocyte-mediated damage, perhaps triggered by a virus infection.

Drug reactions are not uncommon, for example penicillin, sulphonamides, gold salts and penicillamine.

CREST syndrome

CREST syndrome consists of calcinosis, Raynaud's phenomenon, esophagitis, sclerodactyly and telangiectasis. In this condition sclerodermatous skin is confined to the fingers. Vascular and oesophageal involvement may be severe, so this is not a benign disease. Approximately 60% of patients have anti-centromere antibodies but do not have Scl-70.

Eosinophilic fasciitis

This presents clinically with skin oedema and thickening coming on after exercise, usually in older men. Treatment is with steroids although some progress to true scleroderma.

Endocrine organs

Autoimmune disease is divided into organ-specific and non-organ-specific diseases. In organ-specific autoimmunity the damage is directed to cell constituents of one organ only, whereas in non-organ-specific disease the immunological attack is directed against antigenic determinants in several tissues of the body. Many organs have been found to be involved in autoimmune processes.

Autoantibodies in diagnosis The detection of autoantibodies allows a preclinical diagnosis because autoantibodies may be present several years before the disease becomes manifest. Screening is useful in relatives and groups who may be predisposed to disease because of their special characteristics, for example HLA type. In diabetes (see below) autoantibodies may be present many years before clinical symptoms ensue.

The endocrine system
Polyglandular syndrome is where one endocrine disease is present but where autoantibodies to other endocrine glands coexist. There may be clinical damage to more than one endocrine gland producing disease.

Schmidt's syndrome is the association of thyroiditis and adrenalitis. These patients will often also have insulin-dependent diabetes mellitus, which will be associated with islet cell antibodies.

Thyrogastric syndromes highlight the coexistence of thyroid and gastric autoimmunity in the same individual. Pernicious anaemia (PA) is five times more common in patients with thyroid disorders and the corollary is that 10% of PA patients give a history of thyroid disease.

Immunological damage is mediated by antibody directed at cytoplasmic or cell surface antigens, activating complement and binding K cells. Cell antibodies may stimulate the glands. For example, thyroid stimulating immunoglobulin (TSI) binds to the thyroid stimulating hormone (TSH) receptor and mimics the action of TSH itself. Other autoantibodies block the receptor as in some cases of myxoedema. Blocking antibodies as seen in fundal gastritis can inhibit gastric acid secretion. Insulin receptor antibodies can be associated with severe insulin resistance.

Thyroid
The spectrum of thyroid autoimmune disease extends from primary myxoedema at one end to various forms of Hashimoto's thyroiditis with Graves' disease at the other end.

Primary myxoedema is the most common form of spontaneous hypothyroidism in adults. The end stage leads to chronic inflammation of the gland with a female to male ratio of 5:1. More than 70% of the cases are diagnosed over 50 years of age.

Hashimoto's thyroiditis is a common cause of hypothyroidism associated with goitre. All variants have high titres of autoantibodies, although initially the goitre can be associated with normal TSH levels and normal thyroid function. The next stage is clinically compensated hypothyroidism with goitre and raised TSH. Subsequently clinical hypothyroidism results with increased TSH and lowered T4.

Graves' disease is the most common cause of thyrotoxicosis. Peak incidence is between 20 and 40 years of age and it can occur with or without exophthalmos. Radioactive iodine treatment or surgery can be performed after the patient has been prepared with antithyroid drugs.

Diagnosis is by demonstrating autoantibodies to specific thyroid antigens whether surface, cytoplasmic or thyrocyte receptor.

Cytoplasmic autoantibodies are directed against thyroglobulin and TPO autoantigens. 20% of patients have these autoantibodies. In Hashimoto's thyroiditis 95% of patients have anti-TPO antibodies. Microsomal and thyroglobulin antibodies occur in 80% of cases with thyrotoxicosis but are of less diagnostic importance. The disease is caused by thyroid stimulating immunoglobulins (TSI) reacting with the TSH receptor.

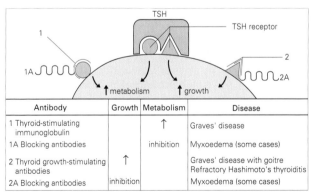

Antibody	Growth	Metabolism	Disease
1 Thyroid-stimulating immunoglobulin		↑	Graves' disease
1A Blocking antibodies		inhibition	Myxoedema (some cases)
2 Thyroid growth-stimulating antibodies	↑		Graves' disease with goitre Refractory Hashimoto's thyroiditis
2A Blocking antibodies	inhibition		Myxoedema (some cases)

Fig. 2.7 Surface of a thyroid cell showing actions of the primary antibodies and autoimmune thyroid diseases. (Adapted from *Essentials of Clinical Immunology* by Chapel and Haeney, Blackwell Scientific Pubs, 1993.)

Stomach

Gastritis occurs in two forms: 1) type A, chronic fundal gastritis; and 2) type B, antral gastritis. These are discussed in the gastroenterological section.

Pancreas: diabetes mellitus

Clinical features are related to altered metabolism and hyperglycaemia due to failure of insulin secretion or decrease in biological function or both. Diabetes mellitus is classified as to whether the patient is insulin dependent (type 1; IDDM) or not dependent (type II; NIDDM) on insulin.

Islet cell antibodies (ICAs) are characteristic of type I IDDM and the disease is the result of autoimmune mechanisms directed against the pancreatic β-cells. ICAs are present in the majority of patients with newly diagnosed type I but not type II diabetes and may be present for years before the onset of disease. Insulitis, lymphocytic infiltration around the islet cells is common, supporting the concept of autoimmune damage.

HLA DR3 or DR4 is present in 90% of Caucasian IDDM compared to 50% in the general population. IDDM susceptibility is even more closely related to the DQ locus.

Heterogeneity among diabetics can be shown by 10% of NIDDM patients having persistent ICA. These subjects tend to progress to overt IDDM.

Insulin autoantibodies (IAA) are described in patients with hypoglycaemia and thyrotoxicosis. The attacks of hypoglycaemia may persist for months and then remit. IgG IAA are found in 30% of newly diagnosed patients and in a proportion of subjects at risk of IDDM – twins or first degree relatives of IDDM subjects. Although IAA is a marker for IDDM, ICA is the best predictor of autoimmune progression.

Adrenal: Addison's disease

Now that tuberculosis destruction of the adrenal is rare most cases (60%) are due to autoimmune processes.

Clinical features are hyperpigmentation, weakness, weight loss and hypoglycaemia, all caused by adrenocortical failure. Mineralocorticoid deficiency leads to renal sodium loss and potassium retention with acidosis.

Autoantibodies can react with all three layers of the adrenal cortex cells. The clinical significance of the different patterns is unknown. Autoantibodies are found mainly in patients with isolated Addison's disease (up to 80%).

The gonads and placenta

Steroid producing cell antibodies cross-react with cells in the ovary, testis and placenta. They have only been detected in sera that also react with adrenal cortex. Whether patients with these antibodies have an increased tendency to premature menopause or infertility is not known for certain.

Pituitary and parathyroid

Autoantibodies in hypopituitarism and hypoparathyroidism are not common but are present more frequently in patients with other autoimmune diseases or polyendocrinopathy.

HLA in autoimmunity

Thyroid cells from patients with Hashimoto's thyroiditis and other thyroid conditions including Graves' disease show HLA-DR molecules on their surface. There is a correlation between HLA-DR expression and the titre of autoantibodies. Class II expression can also be seen in the Islets of Langerhans from newly-diagnosed diabetics. Failure to down-regulate Class II will finally trigger and influence the severity of the autoimmune disease.

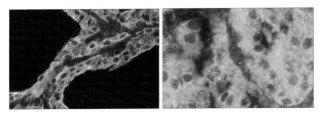

Fig. 2.8 Immunofluorescent staining. (Left) TPO antigen. Unfixed cryostat section of human thyroid stained with serum from Hashimoto's patient. Fluorescence is detected by applying fluorescein isothiocyanate (FITC)-rabbit anti-human Ig, and is restricted to the cytoplasm of the thyroid epithelial cells lining the follicles (×250). (Right) Islet cells – cytoplasmic reactivity. Cryostat section of human (blood group O) pancreas stained with diabetic serum. The antibody reaction is confined to the islet cells. (Latter photograph courtesy of Professor R. Pujol-Borell.)

Kidney

Immune mediated damage to the kidney may be direct, or as a result of a bystander effect. The kidney receives 25% of the cardiac output and the high glomerular capillary pressure increases the susceptibility to circulating factors. DNA may stick preferentially to the glomerular tuft and then may form immune complexes *in situ*. Glomerular cells bear Fc receptors and these may enhance the deposition of immune complexes.

Classification of renal disease can be made on the basis of cases forming part of a more generalized disease such as multisystem vasculitis, where a clear cause can be identified, drug-induced or postinfective, or where the cause is unknown.

Glomerulonephritis (GN)

Aetiology In most cases, no cause can be found. Circulating immune complexes correlate poorly with the presence or absence of GN and activity of disease. Post-streptococcal GN is the best example of acute immune complex nephritis. Chronic immune complex nephritis accounts for more than 80% of cases of human GN. The diagnosis of immune complex GN rests on immunofluorescent findings.

Histopathology findings vary considerably depending on the cause, host response and putative antigen exposure. Deposition of immune complexes may be mainly in the glomerular basement membrane (GBM) or confined to the mesangium. The size of the complexes is important in their localization; an interrupted, granular pattern (punctate) is typical of immune complex deposition in comparison to the smooth anti-GBM antibodies found in Goodpasture's syndrome (Fig. 2.9).

Clinical presentation does not correlate with the histological appearances. Proteinuria is associated with the loss of glomerular polyanions and foot process fusion.

Treatment is supportive. Infection and hypertension must be treated. Hypotension and oliguria in nephrotic syndrome may be helped by albumin infusions. In renal failure, a low protein diet may protect the surviving glomeruli.

Goodpasture's syndrome

Anti-glomerular basement membrane antibody-mediated GN is a severe and often fulminating disease. Antibodies directed against the GBM and alveolar basement membrane in the lungs leads to a rapidly progressive nephritis and lung haemorrhage. Autoantibodies may be triggered by a virus or by exposure to hydrocarbon fumes in susceptible individuals (HLA-DR2). This clinical picture can also occur in multisystem disorders such as SLE or polyarteritis nodosa.

Immunofluorescence shows linear deposition of IgG quite different to the punctate pattern seem in immune complex disease. Antibody eluted from the kidneys of patients with Goodpasture's syndrome reproduce glomerular damage when injected into monkeys. Anti-GBM nephritis can recur in a renal allograft if circulating anti-GBM antibodies are still present.

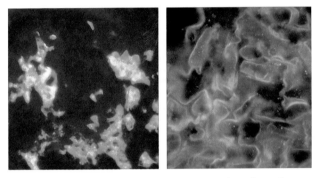

Fig. 2.9 Immunofluorescence study of immune complexes in autoimmune disease. These renal sections compare a patient with systemic lupus erythematosus (type III hypersensitivity) on the left and a patient with Goodpasture's syndrome (type II hypersensitivity) on the right. In each case the antibody was detected with fluorescent anti-IgG. Complexes, formed in the blood and deposited in the kidney, form characteristic punctate deposits (left). The anti-basement membrane antibody in Goodpasture's syndrome forms an even layer on the GBM.

Treatment with steroids and immunosuppressive drugs is not very successful. Outcome has been transformed by the addition of intensive plasmapheresis. No recovery of renal function is to be expected in patients with extensive glomerular destruction.

Multisystem vasculitides

In these diseases, renal involvement is common and is also amenable to treatment.

43

Systemic lupus erythematosus Glomerular deposits occurring in the mesangium and subendothelial areas are associated with high levels of autoantibodies. Membranous GN with immune complex deposition at subepithelial sites is a relatively inactive renal lesion in lupus and is associated with low titres of low affinity antibodies. Free DNA can fix to the GBM of mice and can then react with antibodies. The GN in SLE could develop in this way.

Polyarteritis Focal necrotizing GN is seen in the microscopic variety and the prognosis is worse than in SLE. Macroscopic variety of poly-arteritis affects larger blood vessels and is associated with severe hypertension. Renal lesions are usually infarcts and ischaemic lesions.

Antineutrophil cytoplasmic antibody (ANCA) is helpful diagnostically and as a measure of disease activity, reflecting the presence of vasculitis.

Wegener's granulomatosis
Diagnosis is difficult , despite the triad of midline and lung granuloma, glomerulitis and widespread vasculitis. Biopsies may fail to show disease but ANCA is specific.

Bacterial endocarditis
Clinical features are fever, heart murmurs and glomerulonephritis. In acute bacterial endocarditis, the antigen load is high (antigen excess) and the result is a diffuse, proliferative GN with sub-epithelial immune complex deposition.

Subacute bacterial endocarditis (SBE) The infective load is lower and there is a strong antibody response. These patients are in antibody excess and the immune complexes produce a mild and more focal GN. Rheumatoid factor titres with a low C3 and C4 correlate with the presence of GN in endocarditis.

Treatment with antibiotics usually leads to resolution of the GN.

Hepatitis B Membranoproliferative GN occurs in chronic hepatitis B carriers if the e antigen predominates. The complexes can penetrate the GN and produce a membranous lesion. The surface antigen forms complexes that result in a membranoproliferative picture.

Vasculitis of the large vessels is indistinguishable from idiopathic polyarteritis nodosa. This occurs when the patients have a hepatitis B surface antigen excess.

Cryoglobulinaemia occurs where there are large amounts of antibody to the surface antigen. Patients may be misdiagnosed as essential mixed cryoglobulinaema unless tested for hepatitis B.

Tubulointerstitial nephritis

Drugs are usually the cause. Drugs or their metabolites bind to the surface of tubular cells or tubular basement membranes. The drug then acts as a hapten and triggers an immune response. Antibodies and T cells are involved.

Clinical features Onset may be silent, with proteinuria in association with signs of an allergic reaction such as fever, rash and joint pains. Urinalysis may show tubular epithelial cell casts and red cells. Eosinophils may be present. Proteinuria may be heavy, producing a nephrotic syndrome.

Treatment Withdrawal of the drug is essential. Steroids may hasten recovery.

Amyloidosis is the deposition in tissues of a proteinaceous material derived from the polymerization of partially degraded proteins or polypeptides. The basic structure is that of a β-pleated sheet, thus accounting for its unique staining characteristics.

Classification depends on the parent molecules which undergo partial degradation in an attempt at clearance. Polymerization of the fragments produces the amyloid fibrils.

Diagnosis is by biopsy and staining with Congo Red when the fibrils show apple green birefringence under polarized light.

Treatment is unsatisfactory. Well documented cases of regression are rare, unless the underlying cause can be treated. Colchicine can prevent deposition of amyloid in patients with familial Mediterranean fever. Long term survival is limited by an increased incidence of sepsis and by the consequences of cardiac involvement.

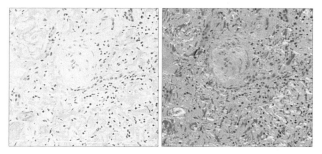

Fig. 2.10 Renal biopsy in amyloidosis. Amyloid deposits demonstrated by Congo red stain (left) show the birefringence typical of amyloid fibrils under polarized light (right).

45

DISEASES OF THE NERVOUS SYSTEM

The central nervous system (CNS) is partly shielded from immune reactions by the low level of lymphocyte migration across brain endothelium and the blood–brain barrier, which excludes large serum molecules such as antibody and complement. Within the CNS, the cells normally have a low capacity to participate in immune reactions – MHC expression is low and the CNS environment itself is suppressive. Nevertheless the CNS contains microglial cells, derived from the mononuclear phagocyte lineage, which can present antigen and secrete cytokines and, when immune reactions do develop, there is a considerable increase in lymphocyte and monocyte inward migration, partial breakdown of the blood–brain barrier and increased expression of MHC molecules.

Multiple sclerosis (MS) is a chronic progressive condition with focal areas of demyelination around venules that disrupt normal nerve conduction. Genetic studies indicate that several genes predispose to the disease. There is also an increased incidence in higher geographic latitudes and evidence that some environmental agent (possibly a virus) encountered in childhood is required for the later development of the disease: it usually develops in the middle years of life. Pathologically, MS shows lymphocyte infiltration in the plaque regions, and breakdown of oligodendrocyte myelin, which is taken up by macrophages. The cerebrospinal fluid (CSF) often contains oligoclonal antibodies, produced locally, but of undetermined specificity. Evidence that MS is an autoimmune disease includes: 1) an MHC disease association with HLA-DR2 with a relative risk of 3.4 and with HLA-DQw1 of 10.5; 2) the specificity of the disease for CNS as opposed to peripheral nervous system (PNS) myelin; 3) various immunological disturbances, such as prolonged expression of IL-2R on activated lymphocytes; and 4) a slight over-representation of myelin-specific T cells in the CSF of MS patients. However no autoantigen or virus has been consistently isolated, and immunosuppression is of limited value. These data imply that the immune response contributes to a multifactorial disease.

Guillain–Barré syndrome is a rapidly developing motor neuropathy, which occurs some weeks after upper respiratory tract infection or vaccination with various viruses. Nerves become infiltrated with lymphocytes and macrophages appear to strip the myelin lamellae of the Schwann cells. It is thought that the infection initiates a T cell-mediated autoimmune reaction directed at the P2 component of PNS myelin.

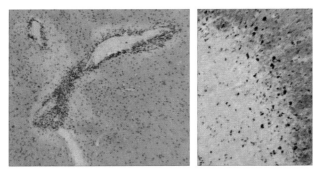

Fig. 2.11 Multiple sclerosis. Perivascular lymphocyte infiltration (left) and demyelinated plaque (right). Courtesy of Drs N. Woodroofe and G.M. Hayes.

Parainfectious encephalomyelitis is an acute disseminated reaction to CNS myelin which occurs after infection or vaccination with various viruses (e.g. vaccinia, measles, herpes zoster, rubella), although virus is not normally detectable in CNS. Perivenous exudates occur, particularly in white matter, with demyelination effected by mononuclear phagocytes. The disease is usually monophasic although a more severe haemorrhagic form may occur. Possibly the viral infection leads to a breakdown in tolerance to myelin, due to alterations in the way myelin is handled by APCs.

Subacute sclerosing panencephalitis (SSPE) is a progressive, fatal disease of children caused by a defective measles virus in CNS, which the immune system cannot clear.

Myasthenia gravis (MG) and Lambert–Eaton syndrome (LES) are conditions in which neuromuscular conduction is blocked. Most MG patients have autoantibodies against the acetylcholine receptor on the motor endplate. These may block conduction directly, but more probably direct antibody and complement-mediated damage to the endplate. Thymoma is a common clinical corollary of MG, and this has suggested that the disease is due to a breakdown in the primary mechanisms by which self-tolerance is maintained. In LES, the autoantibodies are against the nerve terminal at the endplate, interfering with acetylcholine release.

Cerebrospinal fluid immunoglobulin is often raised in diseases of the CNS due to a combination of local Ig synthesis and breakdown of the blood–brain barrier. In viral diseases, much of the antibody is virus specific but in MS the specificity is mostly unknown.

47

THE GUT AND LIVER

Gut

Gut associated lymphoid tissue (GALT) is crucially important, as the gastrointestinal tract is exposed to large amounts of foreign material in the form of dietary and bacterial antigens. An average adult takes in approximately one ton (1000 kg) of food and liquid a year. Oral tolerance with the induction of T suppressor cells and secretory IgA is the key to our ability to handle this antigenic load.

Gastritis can be classified into type A (fundal) and type B (antral) forms. The more common is type A, associated with pernicious anaemia. Both types show chronic atrophic gastritis. In type A the fundus is affected and the antral area spared; the reverse being seen in type B, where there is often the presence of *Helicobacter pylori*. Mucosal lesions in type A must be immunologically mediated, as patients show antibody and lymphoproliferative responses to mucosal antigens.

Clinical features are associated with achlorhydria, failure to secrete intrinsic factor and malabsorption of vitamin B_{12}, leading to pernicious anaemia.

Diagnosis is based on the clinical history and the demonstration of intrinsic factor antibodies. Virtually all the patients with type A fundal gastritis have antiparietal cell antibodies.

Parietal cell (PC) antibodies are directed against the parietal cell canaliculus, the antigen being $H^+K^+ATPase$, which is concerned with acid secretion. Anti-PC antibodies are secondary to autoimmune damage and are detected by immunofluorescence, giving the characteristic pattern.

Intrinsic factor antibodies are of two kinds; one directed against the binding site for B_{12} (blocking antibody), the other against the site that binds to the receptor on the ileal cells (binding antibody). Both lead to failure of B_{12} absorption. It is the presence of intrinsic factor antibodies that makes the diagnosis of pernicious anaemia (PA).

Treatment of PA is with Vitamin B_{12} injections which have to be continued for life. Corticosteroids can have an effect in pernicious anaemia by allowing regeneration of parietal cells leading to more intrinsic factor excretion, thus in turn increasing the absorption of B_{12}. Antral gastritis associated with H. pylori and ulceration can now be treated (with much success) with a proton pump inhibitor and Amoxycillin.

Type	A	B
distribution	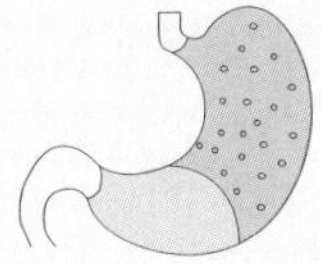	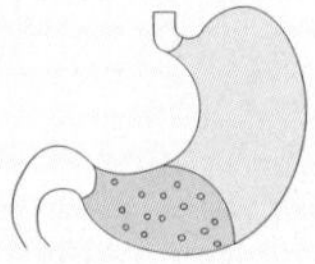
antral inflammation	$\pm$	+++
parietal cell canalicular antibody	+++	$\pm$
intrinsic factor antibody (blocking / binding)	+	−
G cell mass	↑	normal or ↓
serum gastrin	↑	normal
B$_{12}$ absorption	↓	normal

Fig. 2.12 Classification of gastritis, showing the features differentiating the lesion of pernicious anaemia (type A) from gastritis associated with non-immunological conditions (type B).

Food allergy

Clinical features can be confined to the gut with pain, wind, bloating and diarrhoea. Systemic symptoms such as urticaria, arthralgia and mouth ulcers may also be present. Frequently, skin tests and RAST are positive.

Treatment is by avoidance of the culprit food. This is absolutely crucial in patients with nut allergy as laryngeal oedema, asthma, anaphylaxis and deaths are reported each year as a result of nut hypersensitivity. Desensitization is not practicable.

Food intolerance

Clinical presentation may be with migraine, urticaria, irritable bowel, arthralgia, rhinitis, epilepsy, enuresis or hyperactivity. In fact, a very wide variety of clinical conditions can be associated with food intolerance.

Mechanisms of adverse reactions to food are varied and mostly unknown. Some foods contain pharmacologically active substances such as tyramine and some are associated with gut fermentation.

Diagnosis is by elimination diet followed by sequential reintroduction of suspect foods. No laboratory test is as yet reliably diagnostic.

Coeliac disease

Clinical features of coeliac disease vary from vague lethargy and megaloblastic anaemia to the characteristic malabsorption with gastrointestinal tract symptoms.

Gluten sensitivity is the key to the condition but the mechanism is not clear. The three current explanations are not mutually exclusive: 1) hypersensivity to gluten; 2) lectin binding with subsequent damage; and 3) missing enzyme with accumulation of toxic peptides. The disease runs in families and there is a link with HLA-B8 DR3 DQW2. The concordance in identical twins is only 75% so there must be a significant environmental factor.

Diagnosis must be based on jejunal biopsy as the other tests, although helpful, have variable specificity and sensitivity. The jejunum shows the typical villus atrophy with increased intraepithelial lymphocytes expressing the gamma/delta T cell receptor. The atrophy and infiltrate resolve on a gluten-free diet.

Autoantibodies to reticulin, gliadin and endomysium are helpful in screening and there is a reasonable correlation between their presence and the disease.

Treatment is by the avoidance of gluten-containing foods for life. This means not eating most of the foods that contain grains.

Ulcerative colitis (UC) and Crohn's disease

These are chronic inflammatory disorders of the gastrointestinal tract and have a tendency to remit and relapse. UC is confined to the colon whereas Crohn's disease may affect any part of the gut, even including the lips.

Diagnosis of both conditions is made by endoscopy, biopsy and X-ray. Immunological tests do not play any part in the routine assessment of these conditions.

Histopathology is characterized in UC by a dense inflammatory cell infiltrate, crypt abscesses and loss of goblet cells. In Crohn's disease there is also intense cell infiltration but in addition, focal ulceration and granuloma formation.

Systemic signs are similar in UC and Crohn's disease and may be due to immune complex deposition. These consist of aphthous ulcers, iritis, erythema nodosum and arthritis.

HLA-DR is intensively expressed on mucosal epithelial cells in diseased bowel and these cells can act as antigen presenting cells and thus damage can be perpetuated by T cell activation.

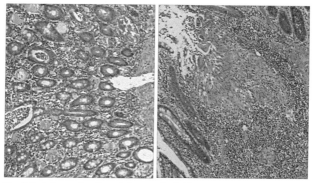

Fig. 2.13 Inflammatory bowel disease. (Left) Histological appearance of ulcerative colitis, showing a dense inflammatory cell infiltrate, crypt abscess formation and loss of goblet cells. (Right) Crohn's disease, showing a dense lymphocytic infiltrate, focal ulceration and granuloma formation.

Sacroiliitis can occur in Crohn's disease and ankylosing spondylitis. In the latter there is a strong association with HLA-B27, which is not seen in Crohn's disease. This suggests that that there are two different aetiologies for the two different types of sacroiliitis.

Food intolerance is a likely aggravating factor in Crohn's disease. Studies with elimination diets show considerable long term benefit when culprit foods are identified and eliminated. Food intolerance does not seem to play a part in ulcerative colitis.

Liver

Hepatitis B

Dane particle. The hepatitis B virion (HBV) is seen on electron microscopy (EM) as the Dane particle, which has a central core containing subscripted DNA polymerase, the e antigen (HBeAg) and the core antigen (HBcAg). The surface coat contains the surface antigen (HBsAg), which was originally described as the 'Australia' antigen. The presence of Dane particles in a serum (detected by EM) is the best indicator of infectivity. Antibody to HBs antigen and HBc antigen indicates previous infection and generally, immunity to HBV.

Transmission of hepatitis B is usually by blood or its products, medical procedures or contaminated needles used by intravenous drug users or tattoo artists. Sexual transmission can also occur. Oral transmission has been demonstrated and HBs antigen has been found in saliva, semen and urine.

Infectivity. Once the virus is attached to the liver cell, viral DNA passes into the host cell nucleus and determines the production of core and surface components. Transcription by DNA polymerase, will produce more viral DNA and hence more infective virions. During this phase surface, core, and e antigens can be found in the blood.

Immune complexes produced during the infective period can produce arthralgia and vasculitis. Dane particles are cleared rapidly and less than 10% of patients with acute hepatitis B progress to chronic liver disease, mainly chronic active hepatitis.

Interferon-α levels are diminished in chronic liver disease secondary to HBV. This could lead to diminished expression of HLA class I antigens, which are necessary for recognition and lytic activity of T cytotoxic cells. Treatment with interferon-α can lead to viral clearance.

Chronic active hepatitis (CAH)

Aetiology. Several causes of CAH are known including autoimmune hepatitis, chronic hepatitis associated with HBs antigen, drugs, α-1 antitrypsin deficiency and Wilson's disease.

Autoimmune hepatitis occurs mainly in young women and is associated with fever, arthralgia and a skin rash. There is a strong association with other autoimmune diseases and the HLA-B8, DR3 haplotype.

Smooth muscle autoantibodies are present in the majority of patients and are mainly antibodies to actin. Other organ and non-organ specific autoantibodies are also present.

Piecemeal necrosis is a feature of liver pathology due to infiltration of the portal tract and liver parenchyma with lymphocytes and plasma cells. The lymphocytes can penetrate the liver substance leading to liver cell death. The inflammation and necrosis subsequently lead to fibrosis and cirrhosis.

Primary biliary cirrhosis (PBC)

Clinical features are pruritis and other features of cholestasis in middle-aged women. Jaundice is a late feature but PBC may be asymptomatic for many years.

Antimitochondrial antibodies and raised IgM are characteristic features. The antigen (M2), a component of pyruvate dehydrogenase complex, is located in the inner membrane of the mitochondrium. These antibodies (anti-M2) are specific for PBC. Antimitochondrial antibodies in other diseases are not against the M2 antigen. Other autoantibodies may be present but are not disease specific.

HLA Class I and II antigens are expressed on epithelial cells of damaged bile ducts but not on normal ducts. Biliary epithelial cells may act as APCs and increased Class I expression may make them more susceptible to cytotoxic T cells.

Treatment is not needed in patients with asymptomatic early PBC. The onset of symptoms or deepening jaundice are bad prognostic features. Unfortunately, no treatment has been convincingly shown to reverse the progression of bile duct damage.

increased:	increased:	decreased:
	IgM (7s)	non-specific cellular
HLA-B8; DR3	C1q, C3	responses
IgG	metabolism	skin test reactions
organ specific disease	immune	lymphocyte function
immune complex symptoms	complexes	

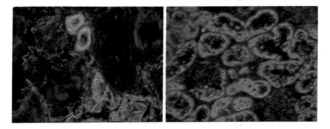

Fig. 2.14 (left) **Chronic active hepatitis:** immunological features include the appearance of smooth muscle antibodies seen here deposited in the arterial walls (×250); (right) **primary biliary cirrhosis:** immunological features include the presence of antimitochondrial antibodies in the serum as shown here by immuno-fluorescence (×250).

THE EYE: OPHTHALMIC CONDITIONS

Episcleritis – a localized, red area of inflammation with lymphocytic infiltration at the corner of the eye. 70% of cases are of unknown cause the rest being associated with connective tissue disorders or herpes zoster infections.

Scleritis may be associated with connective tissue disease and some infections such as herpes zoster, tuberculosis or aspergillus. Immune complexes may deposit leading to complement activation, chemotaxis of polymorphs and possibly autoimmune reactivity. Urgent treatment is needed.

Uveitis is inflammation of the iris, ciliary body and choroid. It can be acute and aggressive in ankylosing spondylitis and Behçet's syndrome. Pus can form in the anterior chamber. Mild forms occur in Reiter's disease and it can be chronic in sarcoidosis and juvenile rheumatoid arthritis.

Retinal vasculitis occurs in a variety of disorders including sarcoid, Behçet's disease, SLE, polyartritis nodosa, Crohn's disease and viral infections.

Allergic disorders
Hay fever conjunctivitis due to grass, tree, weed and ragweed pollen is seasonal. The mechanism is a typical type I hypersensitivity reaction. Similar symptoms can occur in contact lens users who become sensitive to the preservative in the washing solution.

Vernal keratoconjunctivitis is thought to be allergic. Giant papillae occur under the upper lids and local IgE production is increased. Most cases relapse in the spring and summer months. The patients have other atopic disorders, such as asthma, hay fever and eczema.

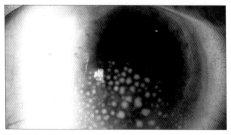

Fig. 2.15 Anterior uveitis. Keratitic precipitates are visible on the corneal endothelium.

a) glaucoma	b) iris-lens adhesion & cataract
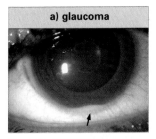	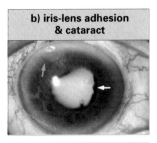

c) retinal pigment epithelium (RPE) disruption	d) macular oedema
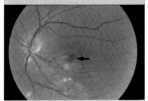	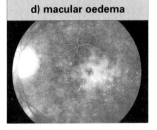

e) pre-retinal collagen	f) leaky retinal vessels
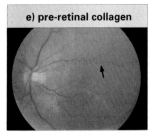	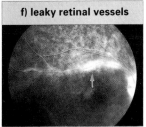

Fig. 2.16 (a) **Secondary glaucoma** due to accumulation of white blood cells in the anterior chamber, forming a hypopyon (arrow) and obstructing aqueous flow. (b) **Iris–lens adhesions** (white arrow) causing iris bombé and secondary angle closure glaucoma, requiring peripheral iridectomy (blue arrow). The lens is cloudy due to cataract. (c) **Disruption of RPE** and secondary growth of a sub-retinal neovascular membrane which has bled (arrow). Pale lesions are seen, presumably due to old histoplasmosis choroiditis. (d) **Macular oedema:** fluorescein dye has leaked at the macula (arrow). (e) **Pre-retinal collagen** causes tangential traction on the retina, seen as tortuous small macular blood vessels (arrowed). (f) **Fluorescein dye leaking** from retinal blood vessels (arrowed) with disturbed endothelial junctions.

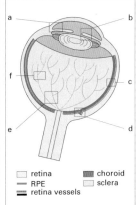

retina	choroid
RPE	sclera
retina vessels	

55

Oral Disorders

The junction between the teeth and the oral mucosa distinguishes the mouth from the rest of the gastrointestinal tract. This junction allows serum proteins to reach the surface and bacteria to reach the alveolus of the mandible via the periodontal membrane.

Dental caries is dental decay caused by bacteria and affects 95% of people in the developed world. Caries does not occur in the absence of bacteria as is shown in germ-free animals. The strongest association with human caries is with *Streptococcus mutans.* This organism is acidogenic and can produce extracellular polysaccharide from sucrose, which is soluble in saliva.

Streptococcus mutans is a likely cause of dental caries, as those with a low incidence of caries have high antibody titres to it. Conversely, those with high caries have a low titre of antibody. These and other studies suggest that serum IgG contributes to protection against caries in man.

Aphthous ulcers

The prevalence is about 10% of the population. A genetic component is shown by a family history being present in 40% and identical twins showing a 90% concordance. HLA studies show a relationship with A2 and B12 (B44). Food allergy can initiate some cases of oral ulceration.

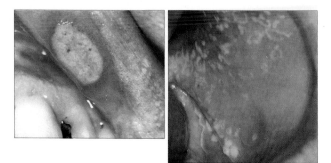

Fig. 2.17 (Left) **Minor aphthous ulceration.** Note the ellipitical shape and defined peri-ulcer erythema. This condition usually affects non-keratinized mucosa. (Right) **Acute pseudomembranous candidiasis (thrush).** There are detachable white plaques on the buccal mucosa which contain fungal hyphae, epithelial cells and polymorphs.

Behçet's syndrome is characterized by recurrent oral ulceration, genital ulcers and uveitis. Skin, vessels, joints, nervous system and gut may also be affected. Antibodies to fetal oral mucosa homogenates and altered complement profiles are seen. HLA-B51 (B5) is raised in all patients, as are DRW52 and DR7. This might be due to linkage disequilibrium with class I genes.

Systemic disease with oral signs

Gastrointestinal diseases such as coeliac disease and ulcerative colitis may present with oral ulceration. Crohn's disease may present as thick rubbery lips or as ulcers.

Oral allergy syndrome presents as itching of the lips and tongue with particular foods. Skin prick tests are frequently positive to both pollens (especially silver birch) and foods.

Skin diseases such as pemphigus and pemphigoid can affect the oral cavity often with overt skin involvement (see 'Skin conditions', pp 62–67).

Pemphigus can lead to ulceration and swelling of the tongue. The typical autoantibody is directed against the intercellular substance in the skin.

Pemphigoid produces bullae, ulcers and desquamation of the gingivae. The typical autoantibody is to epithelial basement membrane.

Connective tissue diseases. Secondary Sjögren's syndrome is characterized by dry eyes (keratoconjunctivitis sicca), dry mouth (xerostomia) and a connective tissue disease.

Wegener's granulomatosis is characterized by necrotizing giant cell granulomas and necrotizing vasculitis. Oral lesions may be the first indication of the disease. ANCA autoantibodies may be diagnostic of this condition.

Oral candidiasis. *Candida* species can be found in the mouths of 40% of normal subjects in quantities up to 800 colony-forming units per ml of saliva. Greatly increased numbers occur in patients with candidiasis where overt oral lesions are seen. Cellular immunity is important and increased frequencies of infection are seen in patients treated with immunosuppressive agents. *Candida* infection is not specifically linked to selective IgA deficiency.

HYPERSENSITIVITY AND AUTOIMMUNITY
RELATED TO INFECTION

Although immunological reactions are generally beneficial, the reaction to an invading organism can also damage the host in a variety of ways. In some instances, this may be difficult to distinguish from the infectious process itself. Antigenic cross-reactivity between pathogen and host may lead to the breakdown of tolerance to host tissues. In other cases antigens from the pathogen may induce hypersensitivity reactions. This is particularly true where high levels of pathogen antigens induce type III reactions (e.g. subacute bacterial endocarditis), but even low levels of antigen release may induce IgE production and type I reactions. Persistent pathogens which evade destruction within tissues often engender chronic immune reactions leading to type IV hypersensitivity reactions and granuloma formation (e.g. in listeriosis or blastomycosis).

Parasitic infections
Hydatid worms release antigen from cysts and this induces IgE formation. Rupture of a cyst leads to a massive release of antigen, which triggers histamine release, which may produce fatal anaphylaxis.

***Ascaris* infestation** also produces high IgE levels, associated with eosinophilic lung infiltrates and asthma as the parasites migrate through the lung. The 'value' of the allergic reaction seems to rest in a lower rate of egg secretion and reduced incidence of anaemia.

***Treponema cruzii* (Chagas' disease)** leads to reduced intestinal mobility and cardiomyopathy with autoantibodies to heart muscle.

Malaria. Quartan malaria is associated with a high antigen load, leading to immune complex formation and deposition in the kidneys and other tissues with resultant type III hypersensitivity reactions.

Schistosomiasis and leishmaniasis both lead to type IV hypersensitivity reactions with formation of granulomata.

Bacterial infections
Rheumatic fever occurs in a minority of patients (<1%) following infection with group A β-haemolytic streptococci. Cross-reactions between bacterial and host antigens lead to autoantibody production, which, in association with tissue inflammation, induces type II mediated hypersensitivity reactions, most damaging against heart valves.

Mycoplasma pneumoniae infection may induce an autoimmune haemolytic anaemia, due to autoantibodies to the Ii blood group.

Klebsiella pneumoniae is thought to trigger ankylosing spondylitis in susceptible individuals via cross-reactivity with the HLA-B27 molecule.

Proteus vulgaris may similarly contribute towards the development of rheumatoid arthritis due to cross-reactivity with HLA-DR2.

Mycobacteria including *Mycobacterium tuberculosis* and *Mycobacterium leprae* both induce type IV hypersensitivity reactions. The lung cavities in tuberculosis and the nerve damage in leprosy are both due to cell-mediated immune reactions against persistent infection. Treatment of leprosy can lead to erythema nodosum leprosum, a type III reaction.

Viral infections

Hepatitis B can induce an immune complex-mediated arteritis in the renal artery, glomerulonephritis or polyarteritis nodosum.

Epstein–Barr virus and hepatitis B can both induce chronic active (lupoid) hepatitis, where the autoantibody is directed against smooth muscle actin. Antibodies to liver and kidney microsomes (LKM) also occur, the antigen being a cytochrome.

Measles virus is associated with a rash, probably due to cell-mediated immunity, as children with defective CMI are prone to infection but do not get rashes. A defective form of measles is responsible for subacute sclerosing panencephalitis, where the high level of measles-specific antibody is unable to clear virus from the CNS.

Fungal infections

Fungi can induce hypersensitivity reactions at the site of infection (e.g. type IV reactions in blastomycosis); other species are responsible for extrinsic allergic alveolitis.

Extrinsic allergic alveolitis (farmer's lung) is due to inhalation of fungal spores (e.g. *Micropolyspora faeni*), which produce immune complexes and type III reactions in the lung, developing over a number of hours after exposure. Symptoms include shortness of breath associated with neutrophil infiltration into the lung.

Aspergillus fumigatus can induce a mixture of type I and III hypersensitivity reactions, producing bronchopulmonary aspergillosis.

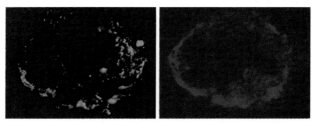

Fig. 2.18 Immune complexes in the renal artery of patient with hepatitis B stained for anti-hepatitis B (left) and anti IgG (right). Courtesy of Dr A. Nowoslawski.

HAEMATOLOGICAL AUTOIMMUNITY

Mechanisms of blood cell destruction. Destruction depends on the class of antibody: both IgG and IgM are involved. Complement needs to be activated and there needs to be interaction with the monocyte–phagocyte system, especially in the spleen.

Intravascular haemolysis is due to complement lysis and is characteristic of IgM antibodies. This is typically seen in ABO incompatible transfusion reactions. Most other alloimmune red cell destruction occurs by extravascular phagocytosis.

Extravascular haemolysis occurs in the tissues and predominantly in the spleen where the bloodstream is slow moving and encourages contact with lining macrophages. Complement components enhance red cell destruction.

Blood group systems. The important blood group antigens in transfusion are those of the ABO system and Rhesus where the D antigen is a strong immunogen (see pp 26–27).

Classification of blood cell antibodies. These may be divided into alloantibodies, autoantibodies and drug-induced antibodies. The specificity of the antibody determines the target of action and the corresponding clinical reaction.

Autoimmune haemolytic anaemia (AIHA) may be primary (no obvious cause) or secondary to pre-existing disease. There is no difference in the autoantibodies in these two groups of patients. AIHA may be due to warm reactive IgG autoantibodies, where in half the patients it is secondary to lymphoma or autoimmune disease, such as SLE or rheumatoid arthritis. Cold reactive IgM autoantibodies can be seen in cold haemagglutinin disease (CHAD), where the haemolytic anaemia is chronic and there is associated Raynaud's phenomenon. Treatment is usually unnecessary, but the patient is advised to stay warm.

Drug-induced immune haemolytic anaemia can be caused by the drug attaching to the red cell and antibodies being formed against the hapten/carrier complex. Antibodies directed against the drug also destroy the red cell. Immune complexes of drug and antibody may be absorbed onto red cells and increase uptake in the spleen. Some drugs trigger an autoimmune reaction by altering the Rhesus (Rh) antigen on the red cell and inducing autoantibodies with Rh specificity. Methlydopa is the drug most frequently implicated.

Autoimmune thrombocytopenia is characterized by a low platelet count and the presence of megakaryocytes in the bone marrow, which excludes primary bone marrow problems. Platelet autoantibodies are absent in 20% of patients. Other conditions should be considered, e.g. post-transfusion purpura and drug-induced thrombocytopenia.

Autoimmune neutropenia is difficult to study because of the limitations of neutrophil serology. It is common in children but not in adults, where neutropenia is associated with other immunological disorders. Neutropenia is associated with SLE and is also seen in Felty's syndrome, where it is accompanied by splenomegaly, high titre rheumatoid factor and rheumatoid arthritis.

Haemolytic disease of the newborn (HDN) affects the fetus and newborn infant when maternal IgG alloantibody crosses the placenta and haemolyses the fetal red cells. ABO isohaemagglutinins are IgM and do not cause HDN (see Fig. 2.19).

Rhesus HDN. Anti-D causes the most severe form of HDN and occurs when a Rh-negative (dd) mother has a Rh(D)-positive fetus. At birth, fetal red cells enter the maternal circulation and can lead to sensitization. ABO incompatibility between mother and fetus reduces the likelihood of sensitization. Rhesus negative mothers are now given anti-D immunoglobulin prophylactically which has considerably reduced the incidence of HDN.

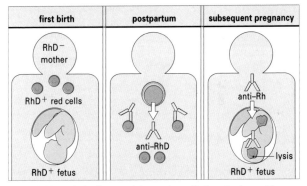

Fig. 2.19 Haemolytic disease of the newborn. Erythrocytes from a Rhesus+ (RhD+) fetus leak into the maternal circulation usually during birth. This stimulates the production of anti-Rh antibody of the IgG class postpartum. During subsequent pregnancies, antibodies are transferred across the placenta into the fetal circulation (IgM antibodies cannot cross the placenta) and can cause red cell destruction.

SKIN CONDITIONS

Many skin diseases show immunological reaction patterns but in the majority the immunological mechanisms are poorly understood.Clearcut immunological reactions in the skin can be classified according to the Gell and Coombs classification. However, some skin diseases, such as atopic eczema, have a complicated immunopathology and this, with those caused by type I hypersensitivity reactions such as urticaria, are described in Chapter 4 (pp 82–95). Hypersensitivity reactions in the skin can be divided into those caused by types II, III and IV reactions.

Blisters are often seen in skin disease and the site of the blisters gives an indication as to cause and mechanism. The majority of lesions are confined to the intra-epidermal or subepidermal site. Subcorneal blisters, just below the stratum corneum are seen in bullous impetigo and some forms of psoriasis. The blisters seen in atopic eczema, pemphigus and Herpes infections are intra-epidermal. Subepidermal blisters are characteristic of pemphigoid but are also seen in dermatitis herpetiformis and linear IgA disease.

Blister level	Condition
Subcorneal	Bullous impetigo, pustular psoriasis
Intra-epidermal	Acute eczema, Herpes simplex/zoster, pemphigus, friction
Subepidermal	Pemphigoid, dermatitis herpetiformis, linear IgA disease, cold and thermal injury, dystrophic epidermolysis bullosa

Pemphigus and pemphigoid

The two main bullous conditions caused by type II mechanisms are organ-specific and autoimmune, namely pemphigus and pemphigoid. Pemphigus is not common but is potentially fatal and both the skin and mucous membranes are affected. Pemphigoid is chronic and is not uncommon in the elderly.

Pemphigus is rare in the UK and occurs in middle-aged people. It is more common in tropical countries affecting adolescents. Before corticosteroid treatment was introduced it was often fatal. The mouth is involved in 90% of patients.

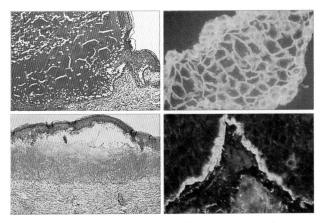

Fig. 2.20 Pemphigus vulgaris. (Upper left) Histological examination shows a characteristic intra-epidermal blister. (Upper right) Immunofluorescence of epithelial fragment showing strong staining of intercellular substance, giving a fish-net appearance. **Pemphigoid.** (Lower left) Bullous pemphigoid: typical histological appearance showing a subepidermal blister. (Courtesy of Dr C Harrington.) (Lower right) Benign mucous membrane pemphigoid: immunofluorescence showing IgG deposition along the basement membrane of the mucosal epithelium.

Aetiology is not known but some drugs can induce the condition possibly by altering mechanisms of recognition of self antigens.

Autoantibodies show an intercellular distribution, the titre of IgG being proportional to disease activity. Pemphigus is a true autoimmune disease, being associated with myasthenia gravis and thymoma and SLE.

Treatment is with high dose corticosteroids (180–360 mg prednisolone daily) and occasionally plasma exchange in addition. Immunosuppresion with azathioprine or cyclophosphamide can be added. Treatment may need to be given for years.

Pemphigoid is relatively common in the UK, mainly affecting people over the age of 60. The most common form is bullous pemphigoid, which affects the limbs and then spreads to the trunk. Oral lesions are uncommon, affecting less than 10% of patients.

Aetiology is unknown but some drugs (e.g. furosemide) have been implicated, as have X-rays and ulraviolet irradiation.

Autoantibodies are directed against the lamina lucida of the basement membrane at the dermoepidermal junction. The titre of IgG antibody does not correlate with disease activity.

Treatment is with corticosteroids but at a much lower dose than that used in pemphigus; 40 mg prednisone daily is usually sufficient.

Diseases caused by type III hypersensitivity

The majority of diseases caused in the skin by type III mechanisms lead to inflammation through deposition of immune complexes in vessel walls of the dermis and subcutaneous fat. The complexes can cause platelet agglutination with the release of vasoactive mediators directly or through mast cell activation with the complement components C3a and C5a.

Dermatitis herpetiformis (DH) presents as subepidermal itchy blisters on the extensor areas of the limbs, shoulders and buttocks. In most patients it is associated with small bowel villus atrophy (coeliac disease) but gastrointestinal symptoms and malabsorption are not common. IgA complexes may not be the cause of the itch in DH as they can be found in the skin of asymptomatic patients.

Diagnosis must be distinguished from eczema, linear Ig disease and scabies. Immunofluorescence shows granular IgA at the dermal papilla and biopsy shows subepidermal bullae. The small bowel can be investigated by jejunal biopsy to show evidence of enteropathy.

Treatment is with dapsone for symptomatic relief and long term gluten-free diet, which will correct both the bowel and skin lesions.

Linear IgA disease is rare and consists of urticarial lesions with blisters. It responds to dapsone. Immunofluorescence shows linear IgA deposits at the basement membrane and may resemble DH or pemphigoid.

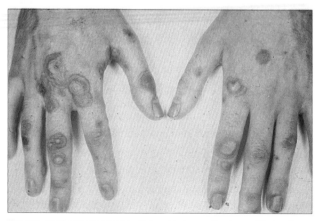

Fig. 2.21 Erythema multiforme with target lesions on the dorsa of the hands.

Allergic vasculitis reflects antigen–antibody reactions producing local perivascular inflammation and purpura. Purpura predominates and presents with a rash over the legs, buttocks and arms. The lesions can ulcerate. Joints and kidneys can be involved and, in severe disease, renal failure can occur. Chronic urticaria can also be caused by this mechanism. Vasculitis as a response to food sensitivity has been reported – tartrazine and azo dyes have been implicated.

Pathology shows prominent leucocytoclastic vasculitis with endothelial swelling, cellular infiltration and thrombosed vessels. Reduced complement levels, a raised sedimentation rate, abnormal proteins such as cryoglobulins with positive autoantibodies (ANA and rheumatoid factor) are found in some cases.

Histology shows prominent vasculitis with endothelial swelling, cellular infiltration and thrombosed vessels.

Henoch–Schoenlein purpura affects children and adults, often after a virus or bacterial infection with *Streptococcus pyogenes*. The purpura is accompanied by proteinuria, haematuria, gut haemorrhage and arthralgia.

Erythema nodosum (EN) is common and presents with tender red nodules on the shins with resolution in 4 to 6 weeks. There is evidence of vasculitis and the most common causes are streptococcal infections, sarcoidosis, tuberculosis, pregnancy and drugs such as sulphonamides.

Erythema nodosum leprosum occurs during the treatment of leprosy and differs from the more common EN in that nodules only last for a week. The lesions are thought to be due to extravascular immune complex deposition. This is understandable as the antigen (*Mycobacterium leprae*) is already in the skin.

Polyarteritis nodosa (PAN) can be fatal with renal and cardiac involvement. The cause is not known but hepatitis B is involved in a quarter of the patients. The disease process in other forms of vasculitis is more benign but in PAN tends to be progressive.

Erythema multiforme has characteristic target lesions on the arms and legs. There is associated stomatitis, iritis and malaise. Vasculitis is present histologically and the condition follows herpes simplex or *Mycoplasma pneumoniae* infection.

Diseases caused by type IV hypersensitivity

Type IV hypersensitivity is based on antigen–T cell interaction with the release of cytokines which in turn recruits other cells to the site of the reaction. The classic response is the tuberculin reaction and contact allergy. Granulomatous reactions result from continuous stimulation with soluble allergen or responses to insoluble antigen, and are clinically the most important form of delayed hypersensitivity causing many of the effects in diseases which involve T cell immunity.

Allergic contact dermatitis is a common example of a delayed reaction in the skin. In sensitized individuals the hapten applied to the skin combines with epidermal proteins to form a hapten carrier complex which stimulates T cells via Langerhans cells. Cosmetics are a very common cause of allergic reactions in the skin with fragrances, preservatives and dyes being implicated. Nickel in costume jewellery causes allergy at the sites of contact. Contact dermatitis can be associated with many occupations, e.g. cement workers' sensitivity to chromate.

Histology shows $CD4^+$ T cells entering the site as early as 4 hours after the challenge increasing up to 48 hours with $CD8^+$ T cells and Langerhans cells increasing over the same period of time.

Clinical reaction consists of erythema and blisters at the site of contact. Some chemicals will sensitize almost everyone, e.g. 2,4-dinitrochlorobenzene, but fortunately only a small proportion of those exposed will become allergic.

Patch tests with a standard battery of at least 22 allergens on small aluminium discs (Finn chambers) is applied to the back of the subject and read at 48 hours with a further reading 2 days later. Positive reactions are shown by erythema and localized eczematous reactions.

Granulomatous hypersensitivity usually results from the persistence in macrophages of micro-organisms, other particles or immune complexes which the cell is unable to destroy. The result is epithelioid granuloma formation.

Histology is different to a tuberculin reaction, which is usually self-limiting and contains characteristic epithelioid cells. Also seen are multinucleate giant cells, which contain several peripheral nuclei. The granuloma contains a core of epithelioid cells and macrophages with giant cells. A non-immunological granuloma, as is seen with talc or silica, does not contain lymphocytes.

Diseases where granulomatous reactions are prominent are tuberculosis, leprosy, leishmania, deep fungal and helminthic infections and sarcoidosis.

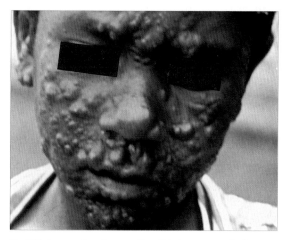

Fig. 2.22 Lepromatous leprosy. The clinical appearance is characterized by marked nodulation of the skin.

Immunodeficiency   3

As the function of the immune system is to protect individuals from infectious pathogens, failure of the immune system often results in increased susceptibility to infections. The types of infectious agents that produce disease in immunodeficient patients are related to the part of the immune system involved. For example, deficiency of complement C3 causes increased susceptibility to bacterial infection, while some T cell deficiencies result in candidiasis or particularly severe infections with herpes viruses. More generally, immunodeficiency describes any identifiable defect in the immune system, whether or not it leads to increased susceptibility to infection. The immunodeficiencies are classified as primary or secondary, where primary immunodeficiency is congenital and secondary immunodeficiency results from external factors, such as infection, toxic compounds, malnutrition, etc.

Primary (congenital) immunodeficiency may be due to abnormalities in genes expressed specifically in lymphocytes and phagocytes, or it may be related to genes that are expressed widely but where the immune system is particularly susceptible to the defect. For example, deficiencies in several enzymes that control nucleoside metabolism are most damaging in lymphocytes, which undergo high rates of division following activation. Gene defects affecting leucocyte development act at different levels in the differentiation pathways (see opposite), with those acting earlier affecting more lineages. However, as the elements of the immune system combine in immune responses, a defect in one section often affects others – T cell deficiencies in particular have wide-ranging effects on B cell and phagocyte functions.

Secondary immunodeficiency may occur in protein/energy malnutrition or where individual nutrients are missing. In particular, low levels of metals (e.g. iron or zinc), vitamins (especially vitamins A and B12), folic acid or pyridoxine all result in impaired immune system function. Some infections lead to reduced or aberrant immune responses, either by overloading the system or because particular leucocyte subsets are targets of infection.

Reticular dysgenesis is a developmental arrest that affects both lymphocytes and granulocytes. Occasionally other lineages may also be affected. The condition causes severe lymphopenia, neutropenia, hypogammaglobulinaemia and rudimentary development of lymphoid tissues. Affected infants die of overwhelming fungal, bacterial and viral infections in the first few months of life.

Severe combined immunodeficiency (SCID) refers to a group of conditions in which both T and B cells are affected. There are both X-linked and autosomal recessive forms, and about 15% are associated with abnormalities of purine metabolism. The disease becomes apparent in the first few months of life and most patients die in early childhood if not treated by engraftment of histocompatible immunocompetent bone marrow.

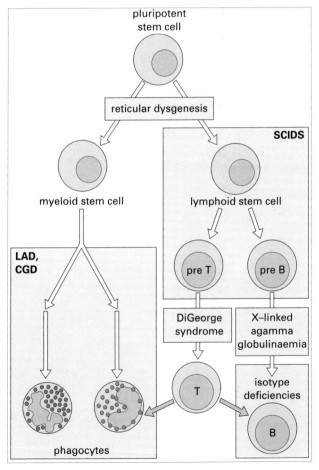

Fig. 3.1 Immunodeficiencies due to defects in lymphocyte and phagocyte development.

LYMPHOID CELL DEFICIENCIES

Deficiencies of lymphoid cells include syndromes such as the SCIDs, which interfere with lymphocyte development, and various enzyme deficiencies that prevent differentiation and/or function of the cells; in conditions such as DiGeorge syndrome the correct environment for T cell development (the thymus) is lacking. These conditions selectively affect the immune system, but there are a number of other conditions, including Wiskott–Aldrich syndrome and ataxia telangiectasia, where abnormalities extend to various other systems of the body. As B cells normally require T cell help to function fully, T cell defects often result in abnormally low antibody responses. This is one of the most readily recognizable consequences of immunodeficiency.

Condition	T cell no.	T cell function	B cell no.	Serum antibodies	Incidence*
XLA, Bruton's syndrome	✓	✓	↓↓	IgG, IgA, IgM↓↓	rare
X–SCID	↓↓	↓	✓	↓	rare
XLP, Duncan's syndrome	✓	↓	✓	✓or↓	rare
X-hyper IgM	✓	↓	✓	IgG↓↓, IgA↓↓, IgM↑	rare
Wiskott–Aldrich syndrome	✓	↓	✓	IgA↑ IgE↑ IgM↓	rare
SCID (Swiss)	↓↓	↓	↓↓	↓↓	rare
ADA deficiency	↓↓	↓↓	↓	↓	very rare
PNP deficiency	↓	↓	✓	✓	very rare
HLA deficiency	✓	↓	✓	poor Ag response	very rare
ataxia telangiectasia	↓	↓	✓	IgE↓, IgA↓, IgG2↓	uncommon
DiGeorge syndrome	↓↓	↓	✓	✓	very rare
IgA deficiency	✓	✓	✓	IgA↓	common

* Approximate incidence: Very rare $<10^{-6}$; rare 10^{-5}–10^{-6}. Uncommon 10^{-4}–10^{-5}; common 10^{-2}–10^{-3}.
Key: ✓ = normal; ↑ = increased; ↓ = decreased or defective.

Fig. 3.2 Immunodeficiencies of lymphocytes.

X-linked immunodeficiencies are a group of rare but genetically distinct conditions, which include X-linked agammaglobulinaemia (XLA), one form of SCID (X-SCID), Wiskott–Aldrich syndrome, X-linked hyper-IgM syndrome and X-linked lymphoproliferative syndrome. Each of these conditions is due to a single gene defect, which specifically affects the immune system. It is now known that hyper-IgM syndrome is due to a deficiency of CD40. The conditions occur in boys, as the normal X chromosome is usually electively used in girls.

X-linked agammaglobulinaemia (XLA, Bruton's disease) causes an arrest in B cell development, so that B cells constitute less than 0.1% of the blood lymphocytes; the residual B cells are immature, with low MHC class II, and high IgM. The lymph nodes are small and lack germinal centres, and immunoglobulins are greatly reduced. IgG is usually present, but at less than 20% of normal values, while IgA and IgM are often undetectable. The effects become apparent after 3 months, when maternally derived antibodies have been catabolized, and the patients develop frequent upper respiratory tract infections. Other complications include severe diarrhoea, encephalitis and arthritis.

X-linked severe combined immunodeficiency (X-SCID) produces reduced or absent T cells, with normal or elevated numbers of B cells. However, antibody levels are low, due to lack of T cell help. Persistent fungal and viral infections develop within the first six months of life.

X-linked lymphoproliferative syndrome (XLP, Duncan's syndrome, Purtilo's syndrome) is characterized by a severe and frequently fatal infectious mononucleosis, in which T cells appear unable to control infection of B cells by Epstein–Barr (EB) virus. Individuals who survive the acute disease have a higher than normal incidence of hypogammaglobulinaemia, aplastic anaemia and lymphomas.

X-linked hyper-IgM syndrome (XHM) shows normal levels of B cells expressing IgM and IgD, but undetectable IgG$^+$ or IgA$^+$ B cells: antibody production to specific protein antigens is usually poor. In addition to bacterial infections, there is an unexpectedly high incidence of pneumocystis infection, which is normally associated with T cell deficiencies. Intermittent neutropenia may also occur. These and other observations suggest a deficit in T cell help to B cells.

Wiskott–Aldrich syndrome consists of thrombocytopenia and various immunological abnormalities, frequently with eczema varying in severity from mild to severe. The primary immunological defect appears to affect T cells, with reduced mitogen responses and low cytotoxic T cell numbers. However there is also low serum IgM and elevated IgA and IgE. A defect in the glycosylation of surface proteins has also been noted. Malignancies occur in 10% of individuals (usually lymphoreticular) and autoimmunity is also common.

Autosomal recessive SCIDs (Swiss type agammaglobulinaemia) affects both B and T cell lineages, but neutrophil numbers are normal, indicating a developmental block affecting the common lymphoid stem cell.

Adenosine deaminase (ADA) deficiency accounts for about 25% of cases of autosomal recessive SCID. The ADA gene encoded on chromosome 20 converts adenosine to inosine in a pathway which scavenges deoxyadenosine. Inhibition of the pathway inhibits nucleic acid synthesis, and interferes with methylation reactions. T cells appear to be highly susceptible to these blocks, possibly because they remain as resting cells for long periods, but may then be required to undergo rapid division following activation.

Purine nucleoside phosphorylase (PNP) deficiency affects the next step along the enzymatic pathway from ADA. T cells numbers are low and responses are reduced, but B cells are present and antibody levels normal.

HLA deficiency (bare lymphocyte syndrome) results in a very rare SCID with normal numbers of T cells and B cells. Individuals with reduced class I expression have few symptoms, but class II deficiency results in a failure to respond to antigens, although the T cells still proliferate in response to mitogens.

Ataxia telangiectasia is an autosomal recessive condition that manifests with ataxia at 2 to 4 years of age. Telangiectases develop over the following years. The immunological abnormalities include reduced T cell numbers and T cell helper functions, including low levels of IgE, IgA and IgG2. Cells of affected individuals often have chromosomal breaks, and the underlying defect appears to be the inability to repair damaged DNA. Patients are susceptible to upper respiratory tract infections but they rarely live to more than 25 years.

Immunoglobulin deficiencies Although many of the SCIDs result in immunoglobulin deficiencies, several less severe deficiencies result in transient or persistent hypogammaglobulinaemia. This may affect one or more immunoglobulin isotypes. The most common single isotype deficiency is of IgA. IgG2 deficiency associates with IgG4 and IgA deficiency and often results in increased susceptibility to upper respiratory tract infections.

IgA deficiency is due to a failure of B cells to secrete IgA; this results in increased susceptibility to infections of the mucosal surfaces, which occurs in about half of the affected individuals. Allergies and many autoimmune diseases have an increased incidence in this condition.

Transient hypogammaglobulinaemia occurs in infancy. There is an extended period following the disappearance of maternal antibodies at 5 months but before the child's antibodies develop to normal levels. The condition is usually self-correcting, with only a slight increase in risk of infection, but some vaccinations are contraindicated.

Common variable immunodeficiency is a group of conditions with no clear pattern of inheritance, which develop in adult life. These result in hypogammaglobulinaemia, with increased risk of infection and a higher incidence of lymphoid neoplasms and autoimmune diseases. Some individuals lack B cells, in others the B cells fail to respond correctly and in others the antibodies are defectively glycosylated.

DiGeorge and Nezelof syndromes both result in thymic hypoplasia due to faulty thymic embryogenesis. This results in reduced T cell numbers and defects in all aspects of cell-mediated immunity. The clinical severity depends on the degree of deficit and partial thymic hypoplasia, which is more common than these syndromes, may correct itself as the mature T cell pools build up with age. Affected children have distinctive features, such as a fish-shaped mouth, wide-set eyes, small ears and a shortened jaw.

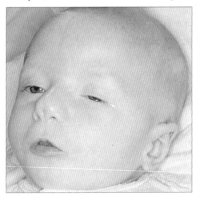

Fig. 3.3 Facial features in DiGeorge syndrome. Courtesy of Prof. A.R. Hayward.

PHAGOCYTE DEFICIENCIES

Mononuclear phagocytes are particularly involved in the control of pyogenic organisms such as staphylococci. Consequently, phagocyte deficiencies often result in infections from such bacteria. Many of the cellular mechanisms of phagocytosis and intracellular killing are used by both neutrophil polymorphs and mononuclear phagocytes, hence many of the deficiencies affect both cell lineages. The processes involved in phagocytosis include: 1) migration from blood vessels into tissue; 2) localization at the inflammatory site, under the direction of chemotactic stimuli; 3) endocytosis of antigens and pathogens, using receptors for carbohydrates, antibody and complement; and 4) intracellular killing of endocytosed pathogens. Phagocyte deficiencies may affect any of these functions.

Leucocyte adhesion deficiency (Lad-1 and Lad-2 syndromes) describes a condition in which phagocyte migration into inflammatory sites is defective. The originally described condition (Lad-1) is due to homozygous deficiency of CD18. This molecule is the common β chain of the leucocyte integrins LFA-1, CR3 and CR4. LFA-1 is present on the surface of phagocytes and activated lymphocytes and binds to ICAM-1 on vascular endothelium at inflammatory sites. This interaction is involved in cell migration into tissues. CR3 is also used by phagocytes to attach to endothelium and both CR3 and CR4 act as receptors for activated complement. Thus cells lacking CD18 migrate less effectively and endocytose complement-opsonized material less well. Recently a second deficiency has been identified (Lad-2). This results in failure to make the carbohydrate Lewis-X, which binds to the selectin group of adhesion molecules. Two of these E-selectin (ELAM-1) and P-selectin are involved in the attachment of leucocytes to endothelium at inflammatory sites.

Lazy leucocyte syndrome is a poorly defined set of conditions in which neutrophil chemotaxis is impaired.

Chediak–Higashi syndrome is a very rare autosomal recessive condition causing aberrant packaging of membrane vesicles. Unsegregated granules in the neutrophils (and also in B cells and natural killer (NK) cells) coalesce and interfere with cell motility. Phagosome/lysosome fusion is also impaired, resulting in delayed killing of endocytosed pathogens.

Neutrophil-specific granule deficiency results in both defective migration due to failure to release chemotractants and also reduces the ability of the cells to kill bacteria.

Chronic granulomatous disease (CGD) appears early in life and is characterized by recurrent infections with catalase-positive organisms,

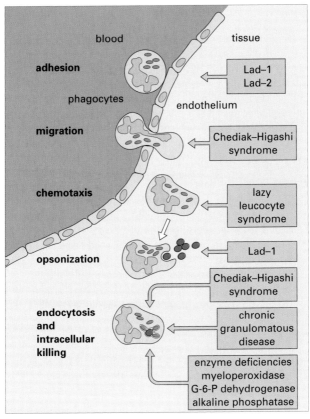

Fig. 3.4 Phagocyte functions and their defects.

such as *Staphylococcus aureus* and *aspergillus*. These often produce disseminated abscesses. The defect is in the killing mechanisms of the phagocytes. Cells of affected individuals produce no respiratory burst after phagocytosis. The most common form is X-linked recessive and is due to neutrophil cytochrome-b deficiency. Less common are autosomal recessive forms of CGD that affect other proteins involved in the cytochrome chain.

Glucose-6-phosphate dehydrogenase deficiency produces a condition clinically comparable to CGD.

Myeloperoxidase deficiency is relatively common, with an incidence of 1 in 2000. The enzyme is normally stored in azurophilic granules of neutrophils and deficiency results in impaired ability to handle fungal infections, particularly candidal infections.

COMPLEMENT DEFICIENCIES

The complement system is a set of serum molecules and associated cell surface receptors involved in control of inflammation. The system can be activated by a variety of microbial products via the 'alternative pathway' or by interactions with antibody/antigen complexes via the 'classical pathway'. These pathways converge on the third component of the system, C3, causing it to become activated to C3b. C3b deposited on membranes, in association with elements of the classical and alternative pathways, can activate the lytic pathway, which lyses plasma membranes. The reactions generate fragments, which perform a variety of important functions. C3 and C4 fragments bind and opsonize bacteria and immune complexes for uptake by neutrophils and mononuclear phagocytes. These cells use complement receptors CR1 and CR3 to bind to the complexes. Ligation of these receptors activates the phagocytes. In man, erythrocytes also express complement receptors and these cells transport complexes to mononuclear phagocytes in liver and spleen. C5a is chemotactic for neutrophils and macrophages and modulates vascular permeability. C5a and C3a trigger mast cell degranulation, thereby modulating local blood supply, vascular permeability and releasing a variety of chemotractants. Examples exist of deficiencies in most of the complement components.

Classical pathway deficiencies (C1, C2 and C4) are associated with autoimmune diseases, particularly systemic lupus erythematosus, although the mechanisms are not understood. C2 deficiency, one of the less rare deficiencies, may also be associated with increased susceptibility to *Haemophilus influenzae* during infancy.

C3 deficiency is very rare but is associated with repeated, life-threatening infections with pyogenic bacteria, which are not opsonized for endocytosis by phagocytes.

Alternative pathway deficiencies (FI and FH) produce conditions clinically similar to C3 deficiency. The absence of these two control proteins leads to unchecked activation of the alternative pathway and hence C3 depletion.

C3 nephritic factor is an autoantibody produced in some patients with glomerulonephritis, which stabilizes the alternative pathway C3 convertase, producing uncontrolled activation of C3, and therefore a functional C3 depletion.

Lytic pathway deficiencies (C5, C6, C7, C8 and C9) are mostly associated with disseminated neisserial infections, although C9 deficiency, which is relatively common is not associated with any particular clinical problem. Autoimmune diseases are also slightly more prevalent than normal.

Paroxysmal nocturnal haemoglobinuria (DAF or HRF deficiency). The complement regulatory proteins decay accelerating factor (DAF) and homologous restriction factor (HRF) are present on cell membranes and limit C3 deposition and lytic pathway activation, respectively. Deficiencies of these components make erythrocytes particularly susceptible to lysis.

Hereditary angioneurotic oedema (HANE, C1inh deficiency) is characterized by recurrent localized attacks of angioedema, affecting the skin or mucosae. This may cause life-threatening airway obstruction. The inherited form is autosomal dominant. C1inh controls several plasma enzymes in addition to C1, and a deficiency leads to uncontrolled local production of kinins. An acquired C1 inhibitor deficiency may accompany some B cell neoplasias.

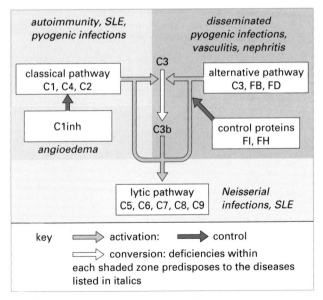

Fig. 3.5 **Complement pathways and deficiencies.**

ACQUIRED IMMUNE DEFICIENCY SYNDROME (AIDS)

AIDS and AIDS-related complex (ARC) are conditions that develop after infection by human immunodeficiency virus (HIV). At present about 50% of individuals develop AIDS within 10 years of HIV infection. The syndrome is characterized by major opportunistic infections, and/or the development of tumours such as Kaposi's sarcoma; some patients also develop neurological symptoms. Following HIV infection there is a transient loss of $CD4^+$ T cells, with acute illness in 10–15% of patients. Some individuals may then develop a persistent generalized lymphadenopathy (PGL), others go on to develop AIDS-related complex (ARC) with a variety of symptoms, such as weight loss, fever, diarrhoea, and opportunistic infections. During these phases $CD4^+$ T cell numbers may be near normal, but as the disease develops into AIDS, there is a progressive fall in CD4 T cells, and reduced ability to withstand infection.

Human immunodeficiency viruses (HIV-1 and HIV-2) The great majority of cases of AIDS are caused by the retrovirus HIV-1, but a related virus, HIV-2 has been identified in Africa. The virus is spread by sexual transmission, infected blood and blood products or transplacentally. HIV uses its surface glycoprotein gp120 to bind and infect cells expressing CD4, primarily T cells, but also macrophages and other antigen-presenting cells.

HIV antigens fall into two main groups, the core antigens gag and pol encode enzymes which are similar between HIV-1 and HIV-2, while the membrane-associated env proteins vary. Core antigens are detectable early after infection, and may also appear as the disease progresses to AIDS.

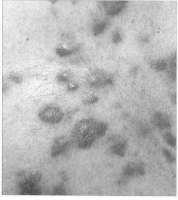

Major opportunist infection

Pneumocystis pneumonia
Chronic cryptosporidiosis
Toxoplasma cerebral abscess
Extraintestinal strongyloidiasis
Isosporiasis
Oesophageal/bronchial candidiasis
Cryptococcosis
Histoplasmosis
Atypical mycobacterial infection
Cytomegalovirus infection
Herpes simplex ulceration or disseminated herpes
Progressive multifocal leucoencephalopathy

Fig. 3.6 Disease markers of AIDS. Kaposi's sarcoma (left).

HIV antibody seroconversion Antibodies are formed to both core and env antigens. IgM precedes IgG antibodies, but there is a period, which may last for several months after infection, before antibodies are detectable.

HIV epidemiology 80–90% of infected individuals in Europe, North America, South Africa and Australia are homosexual or bisexual men, intravenous drug users or have received contaminated blood. In equatorial Africa the disease is equally distributed between men and women, with a pattern of heterosexual transmission. The pattern in South America is intermediate between these two types.

Kaposi's sarcoma produces disseminated nodular lesions and occurs in a minority of AIDS patients. It is associated with HLA-DR5 in some populations.

AIDS neuropathology occurs in a significant minority of cases, sometimes preceding the immunodeficiency. Symptoms range from minor memory defects to severe dementia, and may also include peripheral and autonomic neuropathy and myopathy.

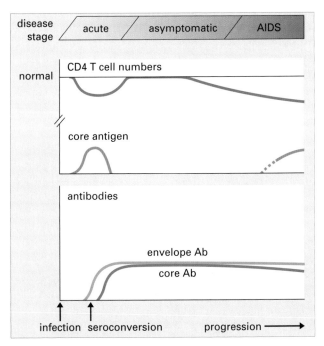

Fig. 3.7 **Serological markers of AIDS infection.**

79

OPPORTUNISTIC INFECTIONS

Many infectious diseases are cleared by the immune system and produce a sterile immunity with long-lasting resistance to reinfection. For other infections immunity may wane with time. A third group of microorganisms, including some bacteria, viruses, fungi and parasites, establishes a permanent occupation of the host. These organisms are normally kept in check by various elements of the immune system and do not produce overt disease. However, in immunodeficient individuals, they represent a permanent danger, because with failure of immunological defences the host–parasite balance is tipped in favour of the parasite. These organisms – referred to as opportunistic infections – act as pathogens in immunocompromised individuals. The range of opportunist infections in such individuals reflects which elements of the immune system are defective. Some of the more common opportunists are listed on this page.

Candida albicans is a saprophytic yeast-like fungus which normally inhabits the gastrointestinal tract. It is associated with T cell deficiencies, including AIDS, but vaginal candidiasis also occurs in about 20% of pregnant women and oral candidiasis (thrush) in around 5% of infants in the first year of life. As an opportunist, *Candida* infects the mucous membranes.

Chronic mucocutaneous candidiasis is a specific immunodeficiency in which the patients appear to be selectively unable to combat *Candida* infections due to failure of the T cells to react to just this pathogen. Infections of mucous membranes, hair, skin and nails may all occur. Endocrine abnormalities may develop later.

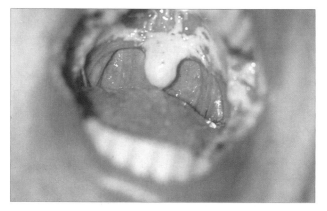

Fig. 3.8 Oral candidiasis in a patient with AIDS.

Fungal opportunist infections In addition to *Candida,* several other fungal infections are associated with T cell immunodeficiency. These include *Nocardia* and *Cryptospora*, which produce pneumonias; the latter may also invade the CNS. The gastrointestinal tract is targetted by *Cryptosporidia*, while disseminated *Aspergillus* can infect any organ, but particularly the CNS.

Opportunistic parasitic infections include *Pneumocystis carinii*, which is the most common pathogen producing pneumonia in AIDS, and *Toxoplasma gondii*, which may produce cysts in the CNS. Both these parasites are associated with T cell deficiencies.

Opportunistic viral infections may be divided into two broad groups: 1) those that affect the skin; and 2) those that develop in other organs. Both are associated with T cell deficiencies. Herpes simplex and herpes zoster both normally lie dormant within neurones, but may reactivate to cause severe localized ulceration. Other viral infections, such as those caused by pox and warts viruses, are more generalized.

Cytomegalovirus (CMV) may affect several organs, producing, for example, pneumonia, encephalitis or infections of the gastrointestinal tract.

Opportunistic bacterial infections are associated with deficiencies in various sectors of the immune system. Mycobacteria may develop in lung, CNS or other internal organs in T cell deficiencies. Staphylococci and streptococci are more often associated with deficiencies of B cells, antibodies and complement (C3) or of macrophage function. However, *Staphylococcus aureus* and other common lung bacteria can produce pneumonia in AIDS.

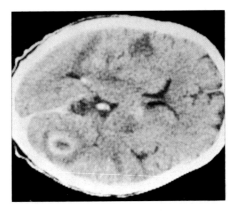

Fig. 3.9 Toxoplasma abscesses in AIDS: CT scan.

Hypersensitivity   4

HYPERSENSITIVITY

When an adaptive response occurs in an exaggerated or inappropriate form leading to tissue damage, the term hypersensitivity is used. The original classification divided reactions into four types (types I, II, III, IV) but clinically these are rarely discrete and may not occur in isolation from each other. The first three types are mediated by antibody and the fourth by T cells and macrophages.

Type I hypersensitivity

The immediacy of the reaction is due to the triggering of IgE sensitized mast cells and basophils to release mediators of inflammation, which produce the clinical effects of allergy. Clinical examples are hay fever, asthma, urticaria, drug allergy and anaphylaxis to bee and wasp venom. The diagnostic skin test with allergen leads to histamine release, which produces a wheal and flare reaction which peaks at 15 minutes and clears by 1 hour unless succeeded by a late phase response.

Type II hypersensitivity

Both type II and III hypersensitivity are caused by IgG and IgM antibodies. The target antigen in type II is part of the surface of a cell or tissue, whereas in type III the antigen is soluble and the antigen/antibody complex causes inflammation wherever it is deposited. Type II mechanisms are important in autoimmunity and transplantation. Antibody bound to a surface antigen recruits phagocytes, activates membrane enzymes and fixes complement. These all produce local tissue damage. Examples of type II reactions are haemolytic disease of the newborn, drug reactions, Goodpasture's syndrome and autoimmunity, e.g. Hashimoto's thyroiditis.

Type III hypersensitivity

Where an antigen persists and soluble immune complexes are formed, diseases such as nephritis, farmer's lung disease, serum sickness and autoimmunity may result. Deposition is determined by the size of the complex, antibody affinity, local blood flow and any pre-existing inflammation. The complexes trigger a variety of inflammatory processes involving complement activation, mast cell degranulation and platelet agglutination. This can induce microthrombi and neutrophil chemotaxis. Skin testing in type III hypersensitivity leads to an Arthus reaction, which is delayed in time compared with a type I response although earlier in onset than type IV skin tests.

Type IV hypersensitivity

Delayed type hypersensitivity is based on T cell-antigen interaction which in turn recruits other cells to the site. The classic responses are the tuberculin reaction and contact allergy. The time course of reactions is more delayed than types I and III, reaching a peak 24–48 hours after injection or contact. This response is used to test sensitivity to micro-organisms such as tuberculosis. With continuous antigenic stimulation, granulomatous reactions occur which cause many of the pathological effects which involve T cell mediated immunity. Contact sensitivity to nickel, chromate, make-up and a number of drugs is important clinically.

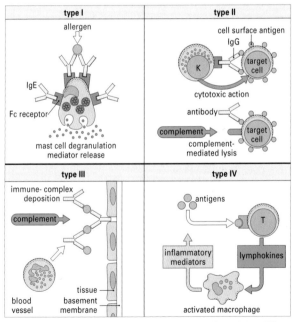

Fig. 4.1 The four types of hypersensitivity reaction. Types I, II and III are mediated by antibodies and Type IV is mediated by cells.

ATOPY

This term describes the tendency of 10–15% of the population to suffer from allergic diseases such as asthma, atopic eczema, hay fever, urticaria and food allergy. There is also a strong family history of similar conditions. Characteristics include a raised serum IgE and positive skin tests to common inhalent and food allergens. Atopy is a convenient umbrella term for those conditions associated with the production of specific IgE following exposure to very low dose allergen.

Fc receptors on mast cells and basophils (FceRI) are high affinity but those on monocytes, macrophages, platelets and B lymphocytes are low affinity (FceRII). Triggering of either of these cell receptors can result in tissue inflammation. New information suggests that monocytes and Langerhans cells also express the high affinity Fc receptor for IgE.

IgE levels are raised in atopics, especially in atopic eczema where they may be astronomical. A raised IgE level aids diagnosis of atopy but a normal level does not exclude it. Specific IgE as measured by a radio-allergo-sorbent-test (RAST) identifies particular allergens that the patient may react to.

Skin prick tests lead to degranulation of mast cells and the release of histamine and the new synthesis of prostaglandins and leukotrienes. The immediate wheal and flare reaction peaks at 15 minutes and can be followed by a late phase reaction 5 to 12 hours later.

The genetics of atopy show that there is a strong family history and where both parents are affected, more than half the offspring become allergic. Environment also plays an important part as is shown by the lack of concordance of allergy in identical twins. Data from environmental pollution suggests that this might be a contributory factor in the increase in allergy in the population.

Asthma

Asthmatics can be divided into intrinsic and extrinsic groups. Both may have a family history of asthma and atopy, have eosinophils and mediators in the sputum and increased IgE.

Allergic reactions can be measured in the lung by respiratory function tests. The immediate response due to histamine release is seen in minutes and is mirrored by a fall in peak expiratory flow rate. The succeeding late phase reaction starts hours later and lasts upto 24

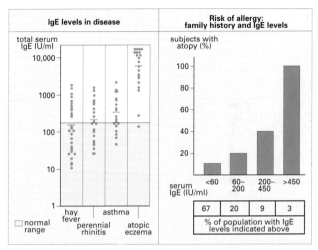

IgE levels in disease	Risk of allergy: family history and IgE levels

Fig. 4.2 (Left) The serum concentration of IgE (around 100 IU/ml) is 10^5 times less than that of IgG (around 10 mg/ml) and comprises less than 0.001% of the total immunoglobulin. Levels in atopic patients are usually raised, especially so in atopic eczema (1 IU = 2 ng). (Right) The higher the level of IgE the greater the likelihood of atopy.

hours. This phase of inflammation with the cellular infiltration is associated with bronchial hyperreactivity.

The immediate reaction can be blocked by sodium cromoglycate, which also blocks the late phase reaction (LPR). Antagonists of prostaglandin (steroids and non-steroidal anti-inflammatory drugs) block the LPR, but not the immediate reaction. The good clinical response to steroids suggests that the LPR is the more clinically important. In a patient of any age who has positive skin tests it is always worth trying sodium cromoglycate or the newer Nedocromil in case inhalent allergic factors are important.

Rhinitis, when limited to the summer or winter is allergic in origin. Pollens cause the summer symptoms and house dust mite those in the winter. Perennial symptoms can be caused by a mixture of both. Food intolerance such as milk, grains or yeast may also cause chronic rhinitis in the absence of positive skin tests.

Aspirin. Sensitivity can be associated with the triad of nasal polyps, asthma and sensitivity to aspirin. Some patients may only experience transient urticaria after taking aspirin for a virus infection. The asthmatic reaction can be very severe and the mechanism is not understood. Mast cell involvement is suggested as is interference with prostoglandin synthetase. Desensitization is possible starting with a small oral dose and then building up.

Bee and wasp allergy is one of the most serious forms of immediate hypersensitivity. Sensitivity to the venom occurs after a number of stings, often when two are experienced with a gap of only a few weeks. Generalized urticaria frequently occurs in children whereas full anaphylactic attacks, and even death can occur in adults. Diagnosis is made on the basis of positive skin tests and positive RAST. Desensitization is indicated if anaphylactic reactions have occurred and is very effective.

Food allergy occurs where the reaction following eating, or even contact, with a food is quick. Swelling of the lips and tongue, generalized urticaria as well as diarrhoea and vomiting may occur. Diagnosis is made on the basis of the history, skin tests and, if necessary, RAST. Occasionally the IgE sensitizes the mucosa of the gastrointestinal tract only and skin tests and RAST are negative.

Oral allergy syndrome causes tingling or swelling of the lips and tongue. There is a cross-reaction between some pollens and foods. Patients with hay fever at Easter time due to silver birch pollen are often sensitive to apples (fresh, not cooked). Other cross-reacting foods are peaches, fruits with pips and some nuts.

Food intolerance is far more common than food allergy. The time interval between eating the food and symptoms is long, hours or even days. This makes the diagnosis difficult. Syndromes strongly associated with food intolerance are irritable bowel, migraine, hyperactivity, urticaria, as well as playing a part in rhinitis, asthma, atopic eczema and arthritis. Diagnosis is made on the basis of an elimination diet followed by reintroduction of foods one at a time.

Skin

In this section, two skin conditions will be mentioned; atopic eczema and urticaria/angioedema. They have the clearest relationship to hypersensitivity and atopy and the role of environmental factors can be clearcut.

Atopic eczema is a puzzle. It is classified as an atopic disorder, being associated with asthma and hay fever, but it has the highest IgE levels of almost any condition except parasitic infections.

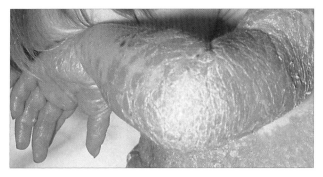

Fig. 4.3 **Extensive atopic eczema.** Courtesy of Dr D. Sharvill.

Patients also have many positive skin tests and a large number of positive RASTs. However, the histology is very similar to allergic contact dermatitis with a lymphocytic infiltration and microvesiculation. This is not the picture of a typical IgE-mediated reaction. There is also evidence of a generalized immune dysregulation.

Hypersensitivity is more likely to be present in the younger patient. Children often have positive skin tests to foods and inhalents. Particular foods can lead to angioedema, urticaria and then acute eczema. The mechanisms for this are not understood. In the older patient, foods do not cause such an immediate reaction and elimination diets are less successful.

Urticaria is an erythematous or oedematous swelling of the dermis or subcutaneous tissue. Angioedema commonly affects the face and lips. Reactions in subjects with food allergy are IgE-mediated and can be associated with diarrhoea and vomiting. Contact urticaria can occur with foods. Common allergens include milk, egg, fish and nuts.

Hereditary angioedema is due to a deficiency of C1 esterase inhibitor or the presence of a dysfunctional protein. In attacks, C1 is activated and C4 and C2 are consumed. Laryngeal oedema and abdominal pain occur. Acute attacks should be treated with fresh frozen plasma or the purified protein. Prophylactic treatment with anabolic steroids induces the enzyme in the heterozygote. Tranexamic acid is also effective in child-bearing women.

RESPIRATORY DISEASE

Lung: protective mechanisms

Protective mechanisms in the lung take different forms: 1) mechanical, where the nose filters out particles, coughing expels mucus and trapped bacteria with the mucociliary escalator continually clearing the bronchi; and 2) non-specific (innate) immune components, which consist of macrophages which comprise 90% of the cell population in the bronchoalveolar lavage (BAL), mast cells, polymorphonuclear leucocytes and complement.

Antigen-specific elements consist of the humoral factors IgA and IgG as well as lymphocytes, which make up 10% of the BAL cell population. The bronchial associated lymphoid tissue (BALT) contains a powerful array of immune cells.

Recurrent respiratory infections may indicate some form of immunodeficiency. A proportion of patients have IgA deficiency and some can have hypogammaglobulinaemia.Others may have HIV-related infections. Any patient with repeated chest infections should be tested for immune function deficits. Chronic infected sputum may be present in patients with immunodeficiency but structural lung damage such as bronchiectasis is also likely to be a cause. In children, cystic fibrosis should be considered.

Asthma

Clinical features are wheezing and variable impairment of lung function when tested over a period of days with a peak flow meter. Sputum and blood eosinophilia may be present.

Precipitating factors may be obvious in that wheezing may be seasonal (caused by pollens in the summer and house dust mite in the winter), associated with the work place or persistent. Non-specific factors such as cold air, exercise or irritants may produce wheezing in someone who already has bronchial hyper-reactivity (BHR).

Skin prick tests are used to show weal and flare reactions of immediate hypersenstivity to a range of allergens in sensitive individuals. Care is needed to correlate the history with the skin tests.

IgE levels and specific IgE antibody titres (e.g. RAST) may add to the clinical data. RAST can be helpful if skin prick tests are not possible because of severe skin disease such as atopic eczema or the taking of antihistamines.

Bronchial provocation testing is important in defining the relevant allergen in occupational asthma, as well as in demonstrating the reversibility of the asthma. It also shows the dual response; namely the immediate asthmatic reaction followed by the late phase reaction.

Late phase reaction (LPR) occurs 5–12 hours after bronchial challenge and is associated with marked cellular infiltration with eosinophils, polymorphs, monocytes and some T-cells. This leads to BHR.

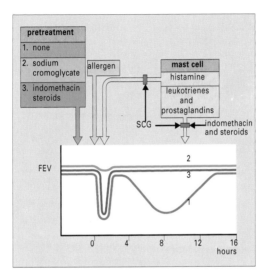

Fig. 4.4 This graph plots the forced expiratory volume (FEV), a measure of lung function, in three groups of individuals prior to and several hours after bronchial provocation with their allergen. In the control (group 1) there is a biphasic (initial and late) bronchial constriction. The initial reaction lasts for 1 hour and is followed by a late phase reaction lasting several hours. Histamine released from degranulating mast cells is thought to be the major mediator of the immediate reaction in man. The other two groups are pretreated differently. Pretreatment with sodium cromoglycate (group 2) inhibits mast cell degranulation thus preventing both early and late phase reactions. Pretreatment with indomethacin or corticosteroids, which block arachidonic acid metabolic pathways, inhibits the late phase reaction but not the immediate reaction (group 3). This implicates leukotrienes and prostaglandins in the development of the late-phase reaction.

Treatment is aimed at removing the cause if possible (e.g. house dust mite, animals) and then treating the symptoms with β-agonists, corticosteroids and sodium cromoglycate (SCG). β-agonists relieve the spasm but do not clear the mucosal inflammation like corticosteroids. SCG is best used prophylactically. Hyposensitization is only possible in the UK in hospitals with resuscitation facilities. Newer low dose vaccines do seem to offer clinical benefit without serious side effects.

Sodium cromoglycate (SCG) blocks the immediate and also the LPR, showing that the LPR requires the degranulation of mast cells for its initiation. Corticosteroids block the LPR alone.

Hay fever

Clinical features are associated with upper respiratory tract symptoms such as sneezing, rhinorrhoea and nasal obstruction following exposure to the allergen (e.g. grass in the summer and house dust mite in the winter). Chronic mucosal inflammation following an allergic insult can lead to secondary sinusitis and secretory otitis media. A detailed clinical history is important.

Diagnostic tests include skin prick tests and measurement of total and specific IgE. In some patients specific IgE may only be found secreted in the nasal mucosa with skin testing and RAST being negative.

Treatment with antihistamines and topical corticosteroid spray is usually effective. Occasionally systemic corticosteroids may be needed if symptoms are very severe.

Interstitial pulmonary fibrosis

Diagnosis. Interstitial fibrosis of the alveolar walls with little involvement of the conducting airways has many known causes. Sarcoidosis and cryptogenic fibrosing alveolitis (CFA) are of unknown cause.

Lung biopsy is an important investigation and may establish diagnosis. Transbronchial biopsy yields more tissue but open biopsy is often necessary to provide enough material for study, for example in CFA.

Bronchoalveolar lavage fluid contains fluids and cells from the bronchoalveolar space and the pattern of cells may give a clue as to the cause of the fibrosis. There are increased lymphocytes in sarcoidosis and extrinsic allergic alveolitis and increased neutrophils with eosinophils in CFA.

Granulomatous reactions can occur through type III hypersensitivity reactions where immune complexes are formed in antigen excess leading to chemotaxis for monocytes and macrophages. Accumulation of these cells at the sites of deposition leads to granuloma formation. Type IV delayed hypersensitivity with T cells and activated macrophages can also lead to granulomata with epithelioid and giant cell formation.

Extrinsic allergic alveolitis

Diagnosis is based on the history of inhaled exposure to organic dusts and symptomatic changes consistent with the disease. Clinically the response depends on the nature and intensity of exposure. Farmer's lung and pigeon fancier's lung are common causes of extrinsic allergic alveolitis.

Classification. Acute recurrent alveolitis occurs in those exposed intermittently to high concentrations of antigen, for example farmers going into their barns once a week. Breathlessness and flu-like symptoms start 4–6 hours after exposure associated with nodular shadowings on X-ray, restrictive lung function pattern and impaired gas transfer. Some patients exposed continuously to high levels of antigen develop aggressive symptoms which may produce a chronic alveolitis.

Precipitating antibodies are a consistent feature in symptomatic patients. However, some asymptomatic exposed subjects can also have precipitins but no evidence of disease.

Histopathology shows diffuse infiltrates of lymphocytes, macrophages and plasma cells with poorly formed granulomata. There is evidence of T cell, B cell and macrophage activation which suggests that this is the more important damaging mechanism than immune complex deposition.

Treatment measures must be based on avoidance of the allergen or at least careful use of filtration masks. Antispasmodics and corticosteroids may also be needed in more severe disease.

Allergic bronchopulmonary aspergillosis

Diagnosis is based on the association of asthma with pulmonary infiltrates and eosinophilia. There is also proximal bronchiectasis and permanent X-ray changes may occur early in the disease.

Aspergillus-specific IgE and IgG antibodies are raised and the patients give positive immediate skin prick tests and also have precipitating antibodies.

Treatment is with oral corticosteroids which control the inflammatory mechanisms responsible for the tissue damage and bronchiectasis. On occasions, the newer imidazole compounds may be helpful.

Adult respiratory distress syndrome (ARDS)

Mortality rate is 50–70% with non-cardiac pulmonary oedema. Pulmonary fibrosis may occur in those who recover.

Endotoxin activation is important and occurs in septicaemia, trauma, aspiration and with some drugs.

Tumour necrosis factor (TNF) is raised in the bronchoalveolar lavage and this up-regulates adhesion molecules on capillary endothelium (ELAM and ICAM-1).

Treatment with antibodies to endotoxin is not effective but the use of monoclonal antibodies against TNF may be helpful. More recently oxypentifylline (Trental) has been effective in treating these patients by reducing the levels of TNF.

Granulomatous diseases

Granuloma formation is seen in many lung disorders and many different mechanisms may be involved. Whatever the mechanism, persistence of the agent is required whether bacterial (e.g.TB) or inert particle (e.g. beryllium).

Pulmonary fibrosis in TB was frequently found at the site of disease activity. With effective chemotherapy it is less common. However, it occurs in about 20% of cases with pulmonary sarcoidosis. Fibrosis depends on specific macrophage activation.

Tuberculosis

Immune response to *Mycobacterium tuberculosis* will govern the extent of the disease. Patients with strong T cell immunity tend to have localized tuberculosis and respond well to chemotherapy. Those who develop widespread miliary TB often have poor cell-mediated immune reactions as shown by skin test reactions and lymphoproliferation *in vitro*. Patients with poor T cell function, e.g. AIDS, are very susceptible to mycobacterial infections.

BCG immunization. BCG is an attenuated strain of *Mycobacterium tuberculosis* used for immunization. Its use has greatly reduced the incidence of the infection. The protection rate is over 80% in the UK, although there is striking geographical and genetic variation.

Sarcoidosis

This is a generalized disorder with the major impact on the lungs. The classification is useful in predicting the clinical resolution in individual patients.

Classification depends on the extent of the disease varying from hilar lymphadenopathy (type I), interstitial shadows (type II) to fibrosis (type III). Resolution occurs in 90% of cases with type I disease. Bronchoalveolar lavage shows a lymphocytic alveolitis, predominantly of $CD4^+$ cells. This is seen even in patients where there is no X-ray evidence of pulmonary infiltrates.

Treatment. As the cause is unknown, non-specific therapy with corticosteroids is given for relief of symptoms and where hypercalcaemia and CNS disease is present.

Systemic involvement is shown with arthralgia, iritis and erythema nodosum (mostly in females) which can be a presenting feature.

Pulmonary eosinophilia

Clinical features are pulmonary eosinophil infiltrates often associated with blood eosinophilia. Classification depends on the cause.

IgE levels and eosinophil counts are raised in helminth infections and especially in allergic bronchopulmonary mycoses.

Tropical eosinophilia is the most important worldwide cause and is associated with microfilariae within the lung parenchyma.
Treatment with low dose steroids usually produces a good response.

Type I
hilar lymphadenopathy

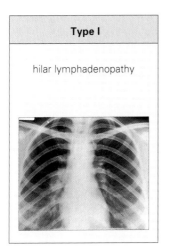

Type II
hilar lymphadenopathy
interstitial shadows

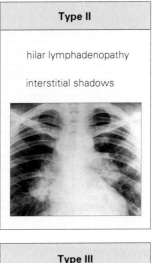

Fig. 4.5 Classification of sarcoidosis. Type I is characterized by hilar node enlargement, usually bilateral. About 90% of Type I patients show spontaneous resolution within 2 years. Type II shows hilar gland enlargement with peripheral lung lesions. Only 60% of those with pulmonary infiltrates clear with the same time scale. Type III is characterized by parenchymal lung lesions only. (Courtesy of Professor M. Turner-Warwick.)

Type III
interstitial shadows
fibrosis

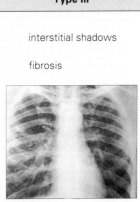

DRUG-INDUCED REACTIONS

There is evidence for an immunological mechanism in some drug reactions, although the signs and symptoms may be due to the underlying disease mechanisms or due to toxic effects. Some drugs can release intracellular mediators by activating the alternative pathway of complement or act directly on the cells themselves – so-called anaphylactoid mechanisms.

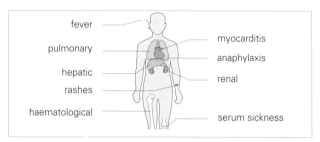

Fig. 4.6 Manifestations of drug hypersensitivity. Several organs are often involved, although presentation may be related to one aspect. Thus, a patient may complain of a rash and be found to have eosinophilia and pyrexia.

Clinical features suggesting drug hypersensitivity include: 1) prior contact with the same agent (or a similar one); 2) reactions occurring with small, non-therapeutic doses; 3) the absence of a dose–response effect; 4) the reaction is not related to pharmacological effect; and 5) only a minority of those exposed are affected. None of these features is absolutely diagnostic for an hypersensitivy reaction. Atopic subjects are not more predisposed to drug allergy.

Manifestations of drug reactions

Skin reactions can be the result of any type of hypersensitivity.

Urticaria can be mediated by type I mechanisms but aspirin sensitivity is also a potent cause. Urticaria is also seen in drug-induced serum sickness which can actually appear after the drug is stopped.

Purpura is a type II cytotoxic reaction against platelets. Antibody and complement are essential for platelet lysis. The classic example of this is the thrombocytopenic purpura due to the 'safe' drug Sedormid.

Vasculitis may be due to immune complex deposition which can be detected by immunofluorescence. In leprosy, erythema nodosum can occur during drug treatment and is due to immune complex deposition containing bacterial antigens released from organisms killed by dapsone.

Contact dermatitis can occur as an occupational disease among production or medical staff or in patients treated with topical preparations containing penicillin, cephalosporin, streptomycin or neomycin.

Blood
Haemolytic anaemia can be due to four distinct mechanisms:

1. Antibody reacts with red-cell-membrane-fixed penicillin and causes a type II reaction.

2. Cephalosporins have structural similarity to penicillin, give a direct antiglobulin reaction but rarely haemolysis.

3. The 'innocent bystander' effect involves a type III drug/antibody complex fixing complement to the red cell membrane causing lysis.

4. The drug modifies the developing red blood cell, which then induces sensitization. Methyldopa, procainamide and mefenamic acid can cause this effect.

Lupus syndrome can be induced by drugs. LE cells, ANF and DAT are the result of the drug forming complexes with cell proteins. Hydralazine-induced lupus appears mainly in slow acetylators and in association with antibodies to single and double stranded DNA.

Agranulocytosis and neutropenia are rarely caused by immuno-logical mechanisms but by toxic effects.

Liver
Jaundice and liver damage due to drugs are probably toxic effects. However, chlorpromazine cholestatic jaundice is accompanied by eosinophilic infiltrates and methyldopa induced hepatic jaundice is associated with inflammation and a mononuclear cell infiltrate.

Kidney
Nephrotic syndrome and oliguric renal failure can be due to type II mechanisms, Goodpasture's syndrome or as a component of serum sickness. D-penicillamine, gold and allopurinol can be associ-ated with immune complex membranous nephropathy.

Diagnosis of drug-induced reactions
Diagnosis is made on the basis of a good history. Difficulties arise because patients are often taking a number of drugs at any one time.

Skin prick tests are helpful in type I hypersensitivity and can be diagnostic with allergy to penicillin, muscle relaxants and local anaesthetics. RAST is available for penicillin.

Patch tests can be very useful in skin reactions due to topical treatment.

Management of drug-induced reactions
Life-threatening reactions need emergency treatment; other mea-sures are necessary where thrombocytopenia or haemolysis occurs. Stoppping the drug is logical even in mild reactions. In difficult clinical situations desensitization may be possible. Where anaphylactic reac-tions occur, the patient should wear a medical bracelet containing the relevant details.

Neoplasias   5

Most leucocyte neoplasias are derived from lymphoid cells. These are broadly differentiated into leukaemias, where the transformed cells are present in blood, and lymphomas, which produce tumour masses in lymphoid tissues. These neoplasias were originally classified by appearance and progression. Now they are usually correlated with cells on the normal lymphocyte differentiation pathways, according to their surface phenotypes (see opposite). Although, these may not be stable in the later stages of disease.

Leukaemias

Acute lymphoblastic leukaemias (ALL) may have the phenotype of either B or T cells. The majority of childhood leukaemias in the 2–6 year age group have early B cell markers such as CD10 or the enzyme TdT, and are often referred to as common ALL. A much smaller group of ALL express markers of mature B cells with surface IgG and Fc receptors. A third group are related to T cells (T-ALL). They are more generally found in older patients, have a tendency to invade secondary lymphoid tissues and usually have a worse prognosis than common ALL.

Chronic myeloid leukaemia (CML) is more common in adults than children. It is thought to develop from transformation of pluripotent stem cells, with the majority of the progeny developing into immature granulocytes. With time (on average 3 years), blockages may occur in the development of these cells, producing an increase in malignancy and often diverting more cells through the lymphocyte lineages. This is referred to as a blast crisis (**CML-BC**).

Chronic lymphocytic leukaemias (CLL) and prolymphocytic leukaemia (**PLL**) may develop from either mature B or mature T cells. In B cell CLL large numbers of immature B cells accumulate in the bone marrow, but do not secrete immunoglobulins, causing a functional impairment in immunity. These cells have abnormally extended lifespans, but the disease course is slow, until it disturbs normal marrow function or blast transformation occurs. Hairy cell leukaemia (**HCL**), so-called because the cells have numerous filamentous projection of the plasma membrane, also expresses mature B cell markers, including Fc receptors, but also has high levels of CD25. This occurs most often in middle-aged men, but is less aggressive than most ALLs.

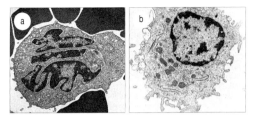

Fig. 5.1 (a) **Sézary cell**; (b) **hairy cell leukaemia**.

Other leukaemias of differentiated lymphocytes include adult T cell leukaemia (**ATL**) which is relatively uncommon in most countries but occurs with a higher incidence in West Africa, the Caribbean and Japan, where it is associated with infection with the human T-cell leukaemia virus HTLV-1. **Sézary syndrome** and **mycosis fungoides** also involve T lineage cells which occur in blood and infiltrate the skin.

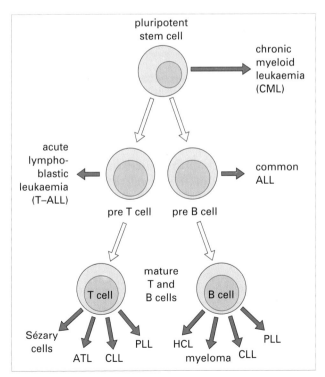

Fig. 5.2 Cellular origins of lymphoid neoplasias.

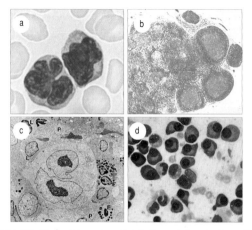

Fig. 5.3 (a) **ATL:** The nuclei are characteristically cerebriform in shape; (b) **NHL:** Section of lymph node showing rounded enlarged follicles with pronounced pale germinal centres and surrounded by a variable mantle zone of small lymphocytes and suppressed (T cell) paracortical areas; (c) **Hodgkin's disease:** Reed–Sternberg cell: eosinophils (e); plasma cells (p); (d) **Multiple myeloma:** Plasma cells in bone marrow.

Hodgkin's disease is a lymphoreticular neoplasia, with cells of various phenotypes present and a significant inflammatory component. It affects primarily the secondary lymphoid tissue, particularly lymph nodes. The critical marker is the Reed–Sternberg cell – large cells with much cytoplasm and a characteristic double nucleus. They are thought to originate from the mononuclear phagocyte lineage. Various proportions of lymphocytes, plasma cells, granulocytes and fibroblasts are also present in the tumour mass. The condition has a bimodal age distribution, with the first peak in young adults and progressive incidence over the age of 50. Younger patients have a better prognosis.

Lymphomas are solid tumours of the lymphoid system, usually derived from cells at a later stage of cell differentiation. In their early stages they do not usually affect bone marrow or haemopoiesis, but autoimmune conditions may develop as normal B cell function falls. Some lymphomas arise from lymphoid follicle centre cells and have the characteristics of centrocytes or centroblasts. A small proportion of lymphomas are lymphoblastic. They have a poorer prognosis and the majority are of T cell origin.

Burkitt's lymphoma is an endemic tumour occurring in tropical Africa, in areas where malaria is prevalent. Sporadic cases occur elsewhere. Epstein–Barr virus transformation of the B cells occurs, which is not controlled by T cells, possibly due to reduced T cell function in the endemic areas.

Waldenstrom's macroglobulinaemia is conceptually similar to myeloma except that the neoplastic cells are abnormal lymphocytes which occupy the secondary lymphoid tissues, rather than plasma cells. They produce IgM which, at high levels, interferes with blood circulation and coagulation.

Myelomas are neoplasias of differentiated B cells. Multiple myeloma usually affects older adults, with large numbers of plasma cells invading the bone and marrow, which may become weakened. The cells produce a monoclonal antibody (a monoclonal gammopathy) which is usually IgG (50%), less commonly IgA or IgM (15–25% each) and occasionally IgD or IgE. Light chains often appear in urine (Bence-Jones proteins). Less frequently, there may be over-production of heavy chains, the most common being α-chain, in alpha-heavy chain disease also called **Mediterranean lymphoma**. This disease is most common in areas of chronic intestinal infections; the gut is massively infiltrated with lymphocytes and plasma cells. Diarrhoea and malabsorption result.

Histiocytosis is a group of neoplasias derived from non-lymphoid cells of the immune system. Many leukaemias that were previously termed histiocytic are now recognized to have lymphocyte markers. The group now includes 'true histiocytic lymphoma', in which the cells express Fc and receptors, and are derived from the mononuclear phagocyte lineage. In histiocytosis X the cells are non-phagocytic and may relate to the dendritic cell lineage.

Chromosome translocation is a regular finding in several of the diseases listed above. The first to be identified was the Philadelphia chromosome, produced by a reciprocal exchange of chromosomes 9 and 22, which occurs in some cases of CML and AML. The gene fusion results in a hybrid tyrosine kinase being produced with increased stability. In other cases, the chromosomal break and rearrangements bring particular oncogenes within the sphere of influence of the promotors which are active in normal lymphocytes. Examples include: 1) Burkitt's lymphoma, where the c-*myc* oncogene associates with the Ig heavy chain locus; 2) 75% of non-Hodgkin's lymphomas have a juxtaposition of the IgH chain locus with a gene BCL-2, a gene involved in protection of cells from apoptosis; and 3) the fusion between TCR-β chain loci and a gene Lyl-1 in T-ALL or between IgH and a gene Pr-1 in B-ALL. Lyl-1 and Pr-1 produce transcription factors that control cell division.

Transplantation   6

Transplantation is increasingly used to treat diseases where failure of individual organs has occurred. The success of engraftment depends on numerous considerations, both technical and immunological. Relevant factors include: 1) the type of donor organ; 2) its availability and condition; 3) the genetic similarity of donor and recipient at histocompatibility loci; 4) whether the recipient has been previously sensitized to any of the donor antigens; 5) the effectiveness of immunosuppression; and 6) the health of the recipient. The following terms are used to describe different types of graft:

Homografts/autografts are from one part of an individual to another. These are the only effective skin grafts available.

Isografts are between genetically identical individuals.

Allografts are between non-identical individuals.

Transplantation antigens (histocompatibility antigens) are allotypically variable molecules, which may be recognized by a recipient's immune system and initiate a graft rejection reaction. Most important is the ABO blood group because the ABO antigens are expressed on many cell types and preformed antibodies in an incompatible recipient lead to rapid graft destruction of, for example, kidney grafts. Also of great relevance are the major and minor histocompatibility loci. The major histocompatibility complex (MHC) is the strongest inducer of T cell-mediated graft rejection reactions. Unfortunately, it is extremely polymorphic, so that it is difficult to obtain perfect donor/recipient matches, except with identical twins. More often a kidney donor will be a sibling or parent, where one of the MHC haplotypes is matched. When using cadaveric organ donors the aim is to have as few MHC mismatches as possible – this is particularly important for the class II DR-loci. There are numerous minor histocompatibility antigens, with more limited degrees of polymorphism, but rejection reactions induced by minor antigens are more readily controlled by immunosuppression than MHC-mismatch induced reactions.

HLA-typing is used to determine the haplotype of donor and recipient MHC loci. The expression of different MHC molecules on the individuals' leucocytes is assessed using haplotype-specific antisera (or more usually monoclonal antibodies), in cytotoxicity or immunofluorescence assays. Antibodies may be used to differentiate class I or class II loci. However, it is also possible to detect class II haplotypes functionally, as lymphocytes recognize allogeneic cells and respond to them by dividing. This is the basis of HLA-typing by the mixed lymphocyte culture reaction (MLC) and the primed lymphocyte typing test (PLT).

Organ	HLA matching	Uses/Comments
cornea	not required for 1st graft	High success rate - cornea is a privileged site. HLA–B and –DR matching for second grafts.
kidney	HLA–B & –DR advantageous	High success rate - treatment of choice for end–stage renal failure.
heart	not usually possible	High success rate - coronary artery disease may complicate graft.
lung	not usually possible	Modest success rate.
liver	not usually possible	Used for hepatoma & biliary atresia. Liver is weakly immunogenic.
skin	essential	Allografts used as temporary cover for burns - replaced by autograft.
endocrine	desirable	Pancreatic islets for type II diabetes. Variable success.
bone marrow	essential	Used in immunodeficiencies, therefore cross-matching or elimination of donor alloreactive cells is required to reduce danger of graft versus host disease.

Fig. 6.1 Areas of clinical tissue transplantation.

GRAFT REJECTION

Privileged organs and privileged sites Like other immune reactions, graft rejection involves sensitization of the recipient to donor antigens followed by recruitment of various effector systems to attack the graft. Some grafts, including cornea, liver and most CNS cell types, are only weakly immunogenic, and hence are described as immunologically privileged. Certain sites on the body are similarly privileged. This is often because they lack a lymphatic drainage, so that donor cells or antigens cannot easily reach the host lymphoid tissues.

Allorecognition covers the ways in which the recipient's T cells may recognize antigens from donor cells. This can occur in several ways. $CD4^+$ T cells have some capacity to recognize allogeneic class II MHC molecules directly, particularly if they partially resemble the recipient's own MHC class II molecules (T cells are selected in the thymus for recognition of self MHC). Alternatively, allogeneic MHC molecules on the surface of a graft cell may present such a dense array of antigen that recipient T cells can still recognize them, even though the individual affinity of binding to T cell antigen receptors is low. A third mechanism for sensitizing the host to graft MHC occurs if the recipient's antigen presenting cells take up graft MHC molecules, process them and present them on their own MHC. This is called indirect allorecognition. Minor histocompatibility antigens must be presented to T cells either by graft MHC molecules or following uptake by recipient antigen presenting cells (APCs).

Passenger cells are leucocytes present in the graft. As they have the potential to migrate into the recipient lymphoid system, and as they may express graft class II and act as APCs, they are particularly effective at sensitizing the recipient. For this reason donor grafts are often treated *ex vivo* (purged) to remove such cells.

Rejection reactions Both antibody-mediated and T-cell mediated immune reactions may be involved in graft rejection. Antibodies may be directed against blood group antigens or MHC antigens. These bind to graft tissue, and cause complement-mediated lysis of the cells or they can direct cytotoxic macrophages or lymphocytes (K cells) to attack the graft. Antibody-mediated reactions are most dangerous, when the donor graft is connected directly to the recipient's vasculature. Cell-mediated graft rejection is directed by $CD4^+$ T cells which can activate macrophages at the graft site. Some $CD4^+$ cells, as well as alloreactive $CD8^+$ T cells may be cytotoxic to graft cells. These types of response are exemplified by the forms of kidney graft rejection, outlined below.

Hyperacute rejection occurs within 1 hour of engraftment and is due to preformed antibodies in the recipient.

Acute rejection occurs 5–21 days after grafting. It is due to sensitization to donor antigens and is mediated by both antibody and/or T cells. If the recipient was previously sensitized to the donor antigens, the response may develop faster (2–5 days) and is called an accelerated reaction.

Chronic rejection develops late after grafting and is due to a breakdown in T cell tolerance to the graft, caused by a disturbance in the graft/host relationship. For example, chronic rejection might be triggered by an infection.

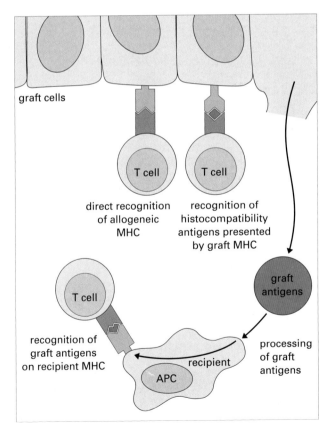

Fig. 6.2 Recognition of graft antigens: allorecognition.

ORGAN TRANSPLANTS

Kidney transplantation is used for end stage renal failure, using relatives or cadavers as donors. Graft survival at one year varies between 70 and 90%, depending on the number of HLA haplotype mismatches (the fewer there are, the higher success rate) and on the centre involved. Although matching of HLA-B and HLA-DR loci is advantageous, matching for HLA-A has no additional benefit when the recipients are treated with the immunosuppressive cyclosporin-A. Moreover, many completely HLA-incompatible grafts survive for extended periods, indicating that the MHC is not the insurmountable barrier to transplantation that was originally supposed. Prior sensitization to donor antigens is also disadvantageous, and transplant centres screen potential recipients regularly for lymphocytotoxic antibodies. The problem is greatest when the recipient has been sensitized to HLA on a previous graft, inducing a broad range of anti-HLA antibodies. Anti-HLA antibodies are also a useful indicator of graft rejection reactions. Individuals who lack HLA-specific antibodies before tranplantation and develop them afterwards have a very low rate of graft survival (12%). Conversely, rare individuals having antibodies before grafting and losing them afterwards have 100% survival. Soluble serum IL-2 receptor is also a marker of rejection.

Heart and heart/lung transplants Although HLA-matching is beneficial in heart and heart/lung transplantation, time does not usually allow this to be done. Graft survival at one year approaches 80% in correctly managed patients. Graft rejection may be assessed by electrocardiographic changes and is confirmed by myocardial biopsy. The myocardium shows enhanced MHC class I expression early during rejection. In this case extra immunosuppressive measures must be started.

Liver transplantation poses great surgical and physiological problems, but the liver is only weakly immunogenic and graft survival at one year exceeds 70%. HLA-matching is usually impractical and has not shown significant benefit. However anti-HLA antibodies in the recipient can selectively damage bile ducts.

Corneal transplantation has been effective for a long period, with a high success rate. The site is partly shielded from immune reactions because it lacks a lymphatic drainage and does not usually possess capillaries. If the site has become vascularized (e.g. following burning) the risk of rejection is greater. HLA-DR matching is beneficial and immunosuppression using steroid eye-drops is also necessary to prevent rejection in most individuals.

Skin grafting is only really feasible as homografts because the skin is highly immunogenic. Nevertheless, it is sometimes necessary to provide a temporary cover following burns, in which case allografts or artificial substitutes are used, to be replaced later by homografts.

Bone marrow transplantation is used in immunodeficiencies, haematological aplasias and to reconstitute the bone marrow of patients who have undergone aggressive therapy for leukaemia. Success rates vary with the disease being treated: ›70% for aplastic anaemia and 10–50% for leukaemias, depending on how advanced they have become. As marrow is highly immunogenic, the best donor is an HLA identical sibling. Failing this, a related donor with one identical haplotype and a partial match on the other chromosome is used, or an HLA-matched unrelated donor. Surprisingly, ABO compatibility is less important, provided red cells are removed from the donor marrow, as stem cells do not express these antigens. The recipient is conditioned with total body irradiation and/or high dose chemical immunosuppression before engraftment to reduce the risk of host versus graft rejection. However, with bone marrow there is also the potential complication of a graft versus host reaction (GvH), as marrow contains mature T cells. For this reason, measures are often taken to deplete the donor marrow of T cells (e.g. by binding to antibody-coated magnetic beads), although these measures usually reduce the success rate of engraftment.

Graft versus host disease (GvHD) is a complication of bone marrow transplantation, where the recipient T cells recognize and react against recipient MHC molecules. Donor alloreactive T cells recruit host effector cells to these sites. The condition usually develops within 4 weeks of transplantation (acute GvHD). The main target organs are the liver (particularly the biliary epithelium), the skin and the gastrointestinal tract. A chronic form may develop later, particularly following acute GvHD. The condition sometimes responds to increased chemotherapy, but in severe cases profound immunosuppression occurs and the patient becomes particularly susceptible to viral opportunist infections.

IMMUNOSUPPRESSION

Immunosuppression is used both for controlling graft rejection reactions and for reducing the severity of immunopathological reactions. In the first case, the aim is usually to prevent sensitization of a recipient to donor antigens: in the second case, therapy is more often directed at immunological effector systems.

Cyclosporin-A and FK506 are fungal compounds that act preferentially at an early stage of T cell activation with various effects, including reduction in cytokine production. Cyclosporin is mostly commonly used in transplantation, although there is increasing evidence that it may be effective in a variety of autoimmune diseases. Less work has been done with FK506: it is effective at lower concentrations and is less nephrotoxic than cyclosporin-A.

Azathioprine and 6-mercaptopurine (6-MP) are purine analogues that act selectively on dividing cells, particularly small lymphocytes. They reduce antibody responses and were formerly used in transplantation, although they naturally also damage other tissues with high rates of cell division, and there is some evidence that 6-MP may cause malignancy. Figure 6.3 compares the effect of different immuno-suppressive regimes on heart transplant patient survival.

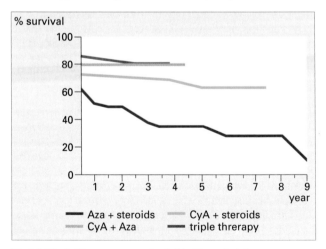

Fig. 6.3 Effect of immunosuppression in heart transplantation.

Anti-lymphocyte antibodies and anti-lymphocyte globulin (ALG) are used to selectively deplete T cells in, for example, transplantation. ALG was originally raised in animals, but has fallen out of use. More recently monoclonal antibodies to leucocyte surface molecules such as CD3 have been used. One problem is that the recipient recognizes the foreign antibodies and makes an immune reaction to them, which limits their long term use. Research is underway to generate human antibodies with the same specificities.

Steroids including corticosteroids and synthetic steroids such as dexamethasone and prednisolone have wide-ranging anti-inflammatory actions; macrophages are particularly sensitive. Steroids also interfere with antigen presentation, and the development of primary immune responses and may reduce circulating T cell numbers.

Total lymphoid irradiation (TLI) acts to damage DNA, indiscriminately. It therefore selectively affects dividing cells. Small lymphocytes are particularly susceptible because they repair DNA inefficiently. Therefore, by dividing the total dose of irradiation over a period of time, it is possible to selectively spare other dividing cell populations. Bone marrow stem cells are also protected during this process by shielding with lead aprons.

Enhancement is a technique used in transplantation to promote tolerance to the graft. The aim is to functionally remove cells which may sensitize the recipient. For example, the graft or the recipient may be treated with antibodies to donor MHC class II molecules. It has also been noted that incompatible blood transfusions, given to a recipient before grafting, unexpectedly enhance graft survival. The mechanism is uncertain, but is thought to be a form of enhancement.

Plasmapheresis is the technique of removing an individual's blood, separating the components, removing the plasma and returning the cellular components. Although the technique has been tried for very many autoimmune diseases, it is only clearly beneficial in a few diseases where autoantibodies of defined specificities are present, including Goodpasture's syndrome, myasthenia gravis and Guillain–Barré syndrome. Its use is more doubtful in generalized autoimmune diseases, where immune complex deposition is important. Plasmapheresis must be used promptly and as an adjunct to other immunosuppression.

Vaccination and Infection 7

Immunization (i.e. vaccination) refers to procedures designed to increase an individual's level of immunity against a particular infectious agent or toxin. Ideally, an immunization should activate the person's own immune recognition system and appropriate effector systems. This is acheived by administering a non-pathogenic form of the antigen and is referred to as active immunization. As strong immune responses take days or weeks to develop, active immunization is normally only useful when given before the real pathogen is encountered. (An exception is rabies vaccine, where the disease is slow to develop and active immunization can induce useful immune responses in time.) However, in some cases the pathogen or antigen is so dangerous that antibodies must be given directly and immediately. This is passive immunization. It is often used to counter the effect of bacterial toxins (e.g. tetanus) or snake venoms. It is also the only approach available in patients with immunodeficiency.

Immune serum globulin (ISG) and immune globulin (IG) are types of antibody preparation used for passive immunization. IG consists of antibodies, directed to a specific pathogen or antigen, used where the pathogen has been identified in the patient. ISG is prepared from pools of plasma with a broad spectrum of antibodies. It is used in individuals with immunodeficiency (particularly hypogammaglobulinaemia), to provide a background level of immunity to a variety of common pathogens and antigens.

Immunity refers to increased resistance to a pathogen, which may be induced by natural exposure or by immunization. The duration of protection varies greatly for different pathogens and with different vaccines. For example, immunity to tetanus toxin, which is primarily dependent on IgG and IgG-producing B cells, may persist for 10 or more years. By contrast, immunity to cholera, which depends on IgA and specific T cell responses, wanes after 3–6 months. Hence immunity depends partly on the site of infection and partly on the type of immune responses effective against it. The second major factor affecting the persistence of immunity is the degree of antigenic variation of the pathogen.

Mucosal immunity refers to protection against infection of mucosal epithelium. This is largely dependent on IgA production and secretion. It is particularly relevant for protection against pathogens that colonize these surfaces and, to a lesser extent, for those that invade the body across these surfaces. Mucosal immunity is induced when the pathogen or vaccine contacts the immune system via the mucosae. For this reason, live attenuated vaccines administered orally, or intranasally are usually more effective at inducing relevant immunity than injections.

Humoral immunity is related to the presence of antibodies in the blood and tissue fluids, particularly IgG. The effectiveness of serum antibody depends on whether the pathogen has a phase in the blood before it reaches its target organ to produce disease. IgG is also very important in protection against bacterial toxins and venoms.

Effector systems are those immune responses that can restrict the spread of infection or eliminate the pathogen. This is determined largely by whether the pathogen is intra- or extracellular. Killing of virally infected cells is mediated by $CD8^+$ T cells. To induce such immunity requires live attenuated vaccines where viral antigens are presented by MHC class I molecules. $CD4^+$ T cells are required to control pathogens that may survive in macrophages; a vaccine must induce cell-mediated immunity. Antibodies of appropriate isotypes (IgG, IgA, etc.) are often effective in controlling pathogen spread or reinfection.

Vaccines are antigen or attenuated pathogen preparations designed to induce protective immunity. It is important, in designing a vaccine to know which type of immunity is relevant to protection – mucosal, humoral or cell-mediated. For antibody induction, the aim is usually to identify critical antigens. Ideally these are antigenically stable. They are usually expressed on the pathogen surface, and antibody against them blocks pathogenicity, e.g. they prevent virus binding to cellular receptors or promote phagocytosis of bacteria, and intracellular killing.

Adjuvants are vehicles for vaccine antigens which enhance the required type of immune response. Alum is the only adjuvant generally approved for use in man. New adjuvants under development include antigen in liposomes and the use of small polymers related to bacterial products.

Antigenic variation concerns the ability of different pathogens to evade immune recognition. This occurs in several ways: 1) some pathogens occur in numerous antigenically different strains, where immunity against one does not protect against another (e.g. colds viruses); 2) some pathogens mutate or recombine sporadically either within an individual or a population (e.g. influenza A); 3) a few pathogens, mostly parasites, have the ability to switch their surface antigens (e.g. African trypanosomes) or disguise themselves using host proteins (e.g. *Schistosoma mansonii*).

Immunogens are the specific antigenic components of a vaccine. These come from different sources for different vaccines (see opposite). The possibilities include: 1) purified antigens or antigen preparations – these may come from the pathogen itself or be produced synthetically by recombinant DNA technology; 2) modified antigens are used where the native antigen is intrinsically dangerous (see below); 3) dead organisms; 4) live attenuated organisms; or 5) antigenically cross-reactive strains of the pathogen.

Toxins (exotoxins and endotoxins) Many bacteria secrete toxic molecules, which may act in the immediate vicinity to promote bacterial spread (e.g. clostridial toxins) or have their major effect on distant organs (e.g. tetanus toxin). These are exotoxins. The endotoxins are cell wall components of some Gram-negative bacteria (*Bordetella pertussis*, *Streptococcus pyogenes* and *Salmonella* species), which can modulate immune responses.

Toxoids are modified exotoxins used in vaccines, which crossreact with the toxin but lack its pathogenicity.

Attenuation is the process by which micro-organisms are rendered less pathogenic for man. Originally, this was done by repeated passage in non-human species or tissue culture (e.g. the BCG attenuated strain of *Mycobacterium tuberculosis*). Current techniques aim specifically to mutate or delete genes that confer virulence on the pathogen, in a way which does not permit reversion, using molecular biological techniques.

Recombinant viruses are a new approach to vaccine development, in which the genes for antigens of pathogens are inserted into infectious but non-pathogenic virus. For example, the gene for the surface protein of hepatitis B has been inserted into the vaccinia virus.

Disease/organism	Immunogen	Duration of protection
Vibrio cholerae	inactivated bacteria	3–6 months
Clostridium diphtheriae	toxoid	→10 years
Haemophilus influenzae	capsular polysaccharide	→4 years
Neisseria meningitidis	capsular polysaccharide	→3 years
Bordetella pertussis	killed bacteria	→6 years
Pneumococcus	capsular polysaccharides	→5 years
Clostridium tetani	toxoid	→10 years
Mycobacterium tuberculosis	BCG, attenuated bacteria	variable
Salmonella typhi	killed bacteria	≥3 years
hepatitis B	surface antigen	→5 years
hepatitis A	killed virus	1 year
measles	attenuated virus	≥15 years
mumps	attenuated virus	≥15 years
poliomyelitis	attenuated virus	>20 years
rabies	inactivated virus	→2 years
rubella	attenuated virus	≥15 years
yellow fever	attenuated virus	≥10 years

Fig. 7.1 Protective effect of vaccines.

Humanized antibodies. One problem with passive immunization (with, for example, immune serum from horse) is that the recipient often develops antibody to the foreign immunoglobin. To counter this, molecular biologists are developing humanized antibodies, where the gene segments for antibody of a particular specificity from another species are inserted into the framework genes for human IgG.

Immunodiagnostics   **8**

The specificity of the antigen/antibody reaction forms the basis of many tests for immunological functions. Antibodies are also used as tools, to detect, quantitate or localize particular antigens in body fluids or tissues. It is therefore important to understand the potentials and limitations of antibodies in these assays.

Epitope is the part of an antigen molecule that binds to any single antigen-combining site. Most antigens have many potential epitopes. However, some epitopes occur on more than one antigen.

Monoclonal and polyclonal antibodies Traditionally, antibodies have been raised by immunizing animals with purified antigens and taking the sera. The antibodies in sera are a mixture of different isotypes with specificity for different epitopes on the antigen. They are derived from many different clones of B cells and hence are polyclonal. Monoclonal antibodies are generated by expanding and immortalizing single clones of B cells, each of which has a defined specificity. Hence the antibodies recognize just one epitope on the antigen, and the antibodies derived from one clone are almost always of a single isotype. Monoclonal antibodies are often generated from mice by fusing B cells with a myelomatous cell line. Human B cells can be transformed with EB virus. It is sometimes thought that monoclonal antibodies have a higher affinity for their antigen, or a higher specificity in recognizing it. Neither of these statements is necessarily so.

Specificity of antibodies depends on the particular system in use, and is essentially subjective. We consider an antibody to be specific when it binds to the antigen in the test material that interests us, but not to other antigens. The specificity of a monoclonal antibody depends on whether the epitope it recognizes is present on any other molecule in the test material. Polyclonal antibodies often have high specificity for a particular antigen because they recognize it via several different epitopes. However, there is a greater chance that one of the component antibodies of a polyclonal mixture will bind to an antigen other than the one to which it was raised, because they share a common epitope. For these reasons, it is essential that antisera are titered out for each type of assay.

Cross-reactivity refers to the observation that a particular antibody can bind to an antigen other than the one that induced its formation. This may be because the epitope occurs on different antigens, or because the cross-reacting antigens have some structural similarity so far as antibody-binding is concerned.

Affinity and avidity Antibody affinity is a measure of the strength of the bond between a single antibody-combining site and an epitope. The avidity is the functional strength of the bond, where more than one interaction may occur.

Antibody titre is the reciprocal of the dilution which is active in the particular assay stated.

Isotypes There are nine different isotypes of antibody in man (i.e. every individual carries a pair of genes for every isotype). These are IgG1, IgG2, IgG3, IgG4, IgM, IgA1, IgA2, IgD and IgE. In mouse, the species from which most useful monoclonal antibodies derive, the isotypes are IgG1, IgG2a, IgG2b, IgG3, IgM, IgA, IgD and IgE. The reagents which detect antibodies vary in their ability to bind to different isotypes and are usually species specific. Reagents used in immunoassays must be selected accordingly.

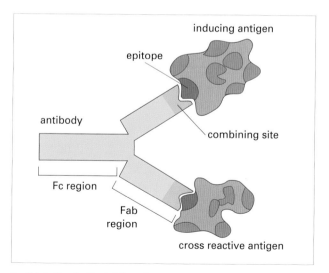

Fig. 8.1 Antigen/antibody interaction.

ASSAYS FOR ANTIGENS AND ANTIBODIES

Radioimmunoassay (RIA) includes a variety of sensitive techniques for measuring antigens or antibodies in body fluids, using a radiolabelled detection system. The assays may be performed in a variety of ways, as illustrated in Fig. 8.2. In each case the reactants are bound to a plastic plate or tube that has been sensitized with the first reagent. Other reactants (antigen or antibody) are added successively, to bind to the plate, and unbound material is washed away at each step. Sometimes staphylococcal protein A or protein G, natural ligands for IgG, are substituted for anti-immunoglobulin reagents. The steps for five typical types of assay are shown in Fig.8.2, where the reactant under investigation is shaded darker.

Competition RIA is used to quantitate antigens. The test antigen competes with a labelled antigen, for the limiting number of binding sites available on an antibody coated tube. The more test antigen present, the less labelled antigen binds.

Direct binding RIA is used to detect antibodies to specific antigens in serum, CSF or other fluids. The antigen is bound to the plate, and antibodies that have bound to it may be detected using a radiolabelled anti-antibody. By using an isotype-specific third layer, specific antibodies of different classes or subclasses can be identified.

Capture RIA is a technique where one antibody is used to capture a particular antigen from solution and another one is used to detect it. Obviously the two antibodies must bind at different sites on the antigen. This technique is used to measure antibodies, where the antibody to be detected acts in effect as the antigen in the assay, and is captured by an anti-antibody. In this case it is possible to substitute radiolabelled antigen in the third layer, so that only captured antibodies with that specificity are measured.

Sandwich RIA is used to detect antibodies in systems where the test antibody acts as a bridge between labelled and unlabelled antigen. Labelled antigen only binds if antibodies of the right specificity form the bridge.

Immunoradiometric assay (IRMA) detects specific antigens. Excess radiolabelled antibody is added to the test solution and any antigen present will bind to it. The residual unbound antibody is then removed with a solid phase antigen. The labelled antibody remaining in solution is proportional to the amount of the original test antigen.

114

Enzyme linked immunoabsorbent assays (ELISA) are a widely used group of techniques for detecting antigen and antibodies. The principles are entirely analagous to those of radioimmunoassays (Fig. 8.2) except that an enzyme is conjugated to the detection system rather than a radioactive molecule. Typical enzymes used are peroxidase, alkaline phosphatase and 2-galactosidase. These can be used to generate coloured reaction products from colourless substrates (chromogens). Colour density is proportional to the amount of reactant under investigation. These assays are more convenient than RIA, but usually less sensitive.

Farr assay uses radiolabelled antigens, which bind to and detect specific antibody in solution. The antigen/antibody complexes are precipitated with, for example, protein A or by physicochemical means (e.g. ammonium sulphate). The radioactive antigen in the precipitate is then measured.

Assay		Steps
competition assay	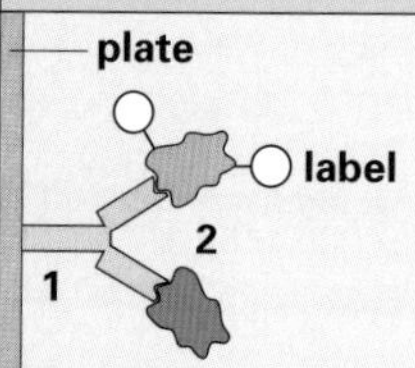	1 specific antibody 2 test antigen plus labelled antigen
direct binding assay	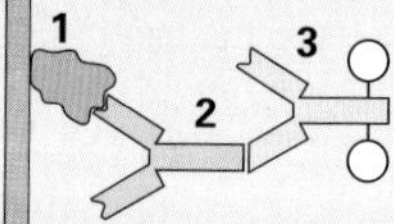	1 antigen 2 test antibody 3 labelled anti-antibody
capture assay	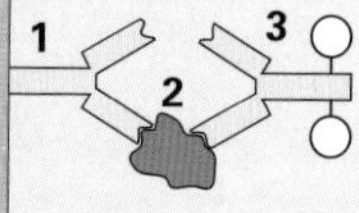	1 capture antibody 2 test antigen 3 labelled antibody
capture assay	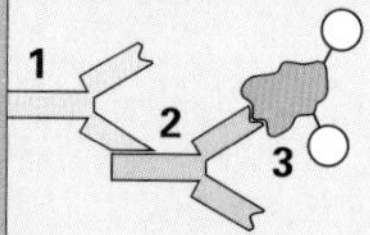	1 capture anti-antibody 2 test antibody 3 labelled antigen
sandwich assay	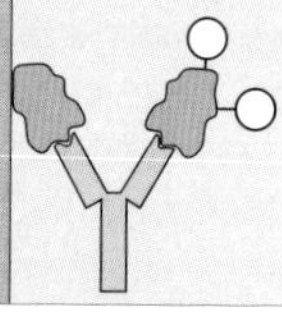	1 antigen 2 test antibody 3 labelled antigen

Fig. 8.2 Radioimmunoassays.

Precipitin reactions are based on the observation that antibodies and antigens may cross-link into large lattices, to form insoluble immune complexes. These precipitates form when the antigen and antibody are present in sufficient amounts, are near equivalence, and when there are enough epitopes available to form a lattice. For this purpose, polyvalent (i.e. polyclonal) antibodies are usually required. Antibodies from some species are better than others in forming precipitates when present in antibody excess. These reactions are used in a variety of assays, in solution or in gels, to quantitate antigens and antibodies. They are much less sensitive than radioimmunoassays or ELISA.

Nephelometry (Turbidimetry) measures immune complexes formed in solution by their ability to scatter laser light. The assay is often used for detection of total antibody by precipitating with anti-immunoglobulin reagents.

Immunodiffusion is used to detect antigens or antibodies in agar gels. The test solutions are placed in wells and diffuse out, towards each other. A precipitin line forms between the wells that contain antigen and the wells that contain antibody. The relationship between different mixtures of antigens or antibodies can be determined by the precipitin pattern.

Counter-current electrophoresis is essentially similar to immunodiffusion, except that an electric current is used to drive the antigen and antibody together. This allows much lower concentrations of antigen or antibody to be detected. The gel opposite (top) shows counter-current electrophoresis using sera from a patient with pigeon fancier's lung (P) on normal serum (N) with antigens from pigeon droppings.

Single radial immunodiffusion (SRID) (Mancini technique) quantitates antigens by allowing them to diffuse outwards from a well into an antibody-containing gel. A precipitin ring forms at equivalence and the area of the ring is proportional to the amount of antigen originally in the well. The technique can be reversed, by diffusing unknown antibody solutions into an antigen-containing gel.

Rocket electrophoresis is essentially similar to SRID, except that the test antigen is moved into the gel by an electric field. Rocket-shaped zones of precipitation form, where the height of rocket is proportional to the antigen concentration. Both this technique and counter-current electrophoresis rely on the antigen and antibody having different electrophoretic mobilities in the gels.

Immune complex assays Immune complexes occur in serum as part of the normal functioning of the immune system. They are usually cleared by phagocytic cells in the spleen and liver, but high, persistent levels may occur in some autoimmune diseases, including systemic lupus erythematosus, rheumatoid arthritis and acute glomerulonephritis. Most complexes in blood (in man) are bound to red cells, which have receptors for them and act as transporters. Some assays to detect immune complexes rely on physicochemical techniques, such as the reduced solubility of complexes in polyethylene glycol (PEG) solutions. Other tests use receptors for bound immunoglobulin such as complement C1q binding or binding to Fc receptors on platelets. Other assays detect fixed complement using molecules such as conglutinin (binds C3b) or receptors on RAJI cells or macrophages. Detection depends on the test employed and is usually of limited use in aiding diagnosis.

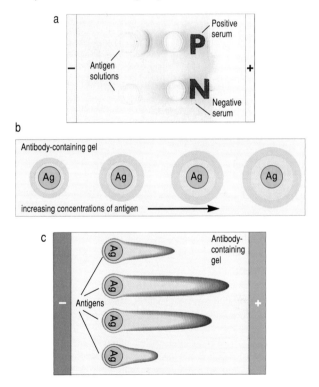

Fig. 8.3 Immunoprecipitation techniques. (a) Counter-current electrophoresis; (b) single radial immunodiffusion; (c) rocket electrophoresis.

Immunocytochemistry and immunohistochemistry are techniques that use antibodies to identify particular antigens on the surface of cells in solution, or on tissue sections respectively. Immunocytochemistry is used to quantitate individual cell populations according to their surface markers (e.g. CD4$^+$ or CD8$^+$ T cells). Immunohistochemistry is used to localize particular cell populations or antigens. These techniques are also used for the identification of autoantibodies, using tissues or cells that contain the presumed autoantigen as substrate. The antibodies are usually identified using enzyme-conjugated antibodies to the original antibody (compare this with ELISA), followed by a chromogen, which deposits an insoluble coloured endproduct on the cell or tissue. The technique is illustrated below in a carcinoma of the breast, infiltrated with CD4$^+$ T cells (left) and CD8$^+$ T cells (right) detected with specific antibodies followed by anti-immunoglobulin coupled to peroxidase.

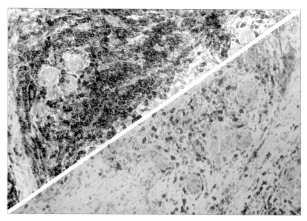

Fig. 8.4 Detection of T cell subsets by immunohistochemistry.

Avidin/biotin reagents are conjugates used for immunocytochemistry and immunofluorescence, which amplify the reactions and increase their specificity.

Immunofluorescence is similar to immunocytochemistry, but uses fluorescent reagents rather than enzyme conjugates. For direct immunofluorescence the antibody is directly coupled to a fluorescent tag – usually fluorescein (green), texas red or rhodamine (red). For indirect immunofluorescence the antibody which binds first is not fluorescent, but it is detected by an anti-immunoglobulin reagent which is. For double immunofluorescence, two different antigens may be detected on the same substrate, by using two independent antibody systems with different colours. Figure 8.5 illustrates the use of immunofluorescence to detect antibodies to thyroglobulin in serum of a patient with Hashimoto's disease on a thyroid section, (left) and anti-nuclear antibodies in SLE on HEP2 cells (right).

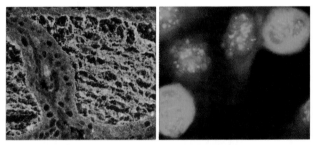

Fig. 8.5 Immunofluorescence to detect autoantibodies.

Flow cytometry and fluorescence analysis A flow cytometer is a device that enumerates cells by counting them individually in a stream. The cells pass through a light beam and the numbers of cells flowing past and (sometimes) the size and granularity of individual cells can be measured, according to how the light is blocked or scattered. Immunofluorescent detection of antigens on the surface of cells in suspension lends itself well to quantitation. The greater the fluorescence, the greater the number of molecules present. A fluorescence analyser (sometimes called a FACS analyser) measures the fluorescence associated with individual cells. As cells can be labelled with two (or even three) different fluorescent reagents, it is possible to determine simultaneously the levels of two surface markers on, for example, a lymphocyte, as well as the cell's size and granularity. This technique is much used for determining the phenotype of particular populations of cells, and the relative proportions of different subpopulations.

Fluorescence activated cell sorter (FACS) is a device that can isolate viable subpopulations of cells according to their surface markers. The machine is based on a fluorescence analyser. The individual cells are stained by immunofluorescence, passed through the analyser and then sorted into different populations according to their fluorescence and hence their surface phenotypes.

Haemagglutination covers a number of techniques for detecting antibodies based on the agglutination of erythrocytes. The antibodies may be directed to the red cell antigens. These occur, for example, in autoimmune haemolytic anaemias, or when an individual has natural or induced antibodies to allogeneic erythrocytes (see page 27, Coombs test). Alternatively, many antigens may be chemically coupled to red cells to detect specific antibodies. The antibodies are serially diluted on plates before addition of the antigen-sensitized erythrocytes. If antibody is present the red cells cross-link and sink as a mat to the bottom of the well, if not they roll down to form a pellet. The technique is as sensitive as ELISA. In the example below sera from eight individuals have been serially diluted, on separate rows of the plate. Wells 11 and 12 contain positive and negative controls respectively. Antigen-sensitised erythrocytes were added to each well. As examples, the individual on row A shows an antibody titre of 1/32, B is negative and E is 1/256.

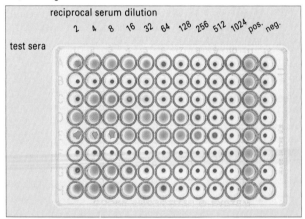

Fig. 8.6 Antibody detection by haemagglutination.

Complement fixation test is used to detect antibodies, by their ability to bind to antigen in solution, form immune complexes and then consume complement molecules. It may similarly be used to detect antigens. The assay is sensitive, but as immune complexes or other complement-consuming molecules may occur in serum anyway, the assay must be rigorously controlled for such artefacts.

Western blotting (immunoblotting) is used to characterize unknown antigens. An antigen mixture is separated by gel electrophoresis: SDS gels separate according to molecular weight; IEF gels according to charge characteristics. The separated proteins are transferred to membranes (blotted) and identified by immunocytochemistry.

MOLECULAR BIOLOGICAL TECHNIQUES

Polymerase chain reaction (PCR) is a technique used to amplify small amounts of DNA or RNA, which can be applied to diverse starting material – cell extracts, tissue sections, autopsy material, etc. Hence, assays can be carried out starting with very small amounts of nucleic acids. The material amplified depends critically on the initial sample so contamination with extraneous DNA must be excluded. The segment of DNA that will be amplified depends on the use of primers that flank the sequences of interest.

Southern blotting is used to detect specific segments of DNA separated in agarose gels and then blotted onto membranes. The blots are hybridized with labelled DNA segments. These attach to complementary sequences on the blot. Depending on the conditions, hybridization can be done at high stringency or low stringency. At high stringency the procedure will tolerate only a low number of base mismatches between the DNA on the blot and the DNA probe. Low stringency tolerates more mismatches. The technique is used, for example, to detect particular DNA haplotypes of polymorphic molecules such as MHC antigens. It is also used in association with restriction fragment length polymorphism (RFLP) analysis for genetic fingerprinting.

Restriction fragment length polymorphism (RFLP) is an older technique for determining variability in DNA from different individuals. Certain bacterial enzymes recognize and cleave DNA at particular sequences. These enzymes cut genomic DNA into fragments of particular sizes, depending on where the specific sequences lie. Different individuals may vary in the number and location of these sequences (polymorphism). This is detected by separating the cleaved DNA on gels and carrying out Southern blotting using probes which bind near to the gene of interest.

Northern blotting is technically similar to Southern blotting but is used to separate and detect RNA, not DNA. The method is useful for determining whether particular species of mRNA are present in test material, i.e. it identifies which genes are being transcribed.

***In situ* hybridization** is a technique used to detect mRNA species expressed in tissue sections. cDNA probes are hybridized to the section *in situ*, showing whether particular genes are transcribed, and also which cell types are transcribing them. For example, it can be used to show transcription of cytokine genes in areas of inflammation. It is particularly useful for identifying which cell type is transcribing a particular gene.

ISOLATION OF CELLS

Ficoll gradients are used to separate leucocytes, particularly lymphocytes from the blood, on the basis of their density. The blood sample is defibrinated, and then diluted before overlaying on Ficoll. The tubes are centrifuged. Red cells and most granulocytes sink through the Ficoll. Lymphocytes and most monocytes float at the interface between the Ficoll and the diluted plasma, and can be removed by aspiration. This fraction constitutes peripheral blood mononuclear cells (PBMCs) used in many assays. The fraction may be further depleted of phagocytes before use. It is also possible to change the concentration (density) of the Ficoll to isolate different populations of leucocytes.

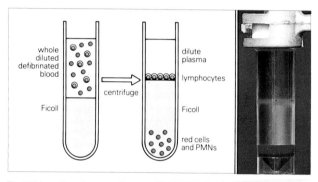

Fig. 8.7 Lymphocyte separation on a Ficoll isopaque gradient.

Rosetting is a technique used to isolate human T cells, which bind to sheep erythrocytes via CD2/LFA-3. The T cells form rosettes with the red cells, making them more dense so that they can be separated by spinning down through Ficoll. The technique may be modified using erythrocytes sensitized with particular antibodies to get other cell populations.

Magnetic beads can be sensitized with antibodies and used to isolate specific populations of lymphocytes. For example, beads sensitized with anti-CD4 will bind to the CD4$^+$ T cell population, which can then be isolated using a magnet.

Adherence to plastic plates can be used to isolate cells. Macrophages and monocytes adhere directly to plastic, but other populations can be separated by applying them to plates sensitized with specific antibodies.

FUNCTIONAL ASSAYS

Assays for lymphocyte function depend on the cell type being investigated. B cell activity is measured by antibody production: T cells are assessed by the ability to proliferate in response to antigen, to secrete cytokines or to act as cytotoxic cells.

Transformation in an immunological context refers to the change from resting cell to blast cell which occurs when lymphocytes are activated by antigen on suitable antigen-presenting cells. This precedes cell division.

Proliferation assays are used to measure whether T cells are present which can respond to antigen. The test lymphocytes are cultured with a population of syngeneic antigen-presenting cells and the antigen. After about 3 days of coculture, radiolabelled nucleic acid precursors are added to the culture (e.g. ^{3}H-thymidine). If proliferating cells are present they take up the precursors. The cell culture is then harvested and the amount of radiolabel incorporated into the cells is measured. High incorporation indicates the presence of responding cells.

Mixed lymphocyte culture/reaction (MLC/MLR) is a proliferation assay used to determine whether T cells are present which respond to allogeneic cells. It may be used as an adjunct to tissue-typing, to determine whether T cells in a potential recipient will react against donor HLA class II molecules. In this case the stimulating antigen is lymphocytes from the donor which have been irradiated so that they themselves cannot proliferate. The stimulating lymphocytes act as both APC and antigen in this assay.

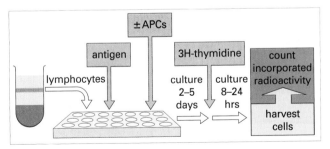

Fig. 8.8 Lymphocyte proliferation assay.

Mixed lymphocyte target interaction (MLTI) is a proliferation assay sometimes used in the study of an individual's anti-tumour response. The patient's lymphocytes are stimulated with irradiated tumour cells.

Cytokine assays Functionally, many cytokines may be assayed according to their ability to permit growth of specific cell lines. For example IL-2 is measured by its ability to induce division of an IL-2-dependent cell line, in a proliferation assay. Many cytokines can also be quantitated by radioimmunoassay or ELISA, with cytokine-specific antibodies. The number of cells producing individual cytokines are measured by a modification of the ELISPOT assay using anti-cytokine antibody.

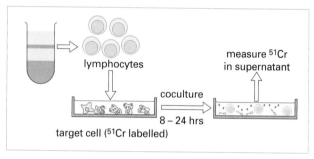

Fig. 8.9 Chromium release assay for cytotoxicity.

Cytotoxicity assays Cytotoxic activity of lymphocytes is measured by coculture with target cells, which have been labelled with, for example, ^{51}Cr. If lymphocytes kill the targets, the chromium is released and the radioactivity released into the culture medium is a measure of cytotoxic activity. Antibody and complement-mediated cytotoxicity can also be measured by chromium release, but may also be carried out more simply by dye exclusion. Certain dyes, including trypan blue and ethidium bromide, are excluded from viable cells. Hence, dead cells can be quantitated microscopically by positive staining.

Plaque forming cell (PFC) assays are used to enumerate individual antibody-producing B cells. The test cells are cocultured with erythrocytes sensitized with antigen (cf haemagglutination). Specific antibody binds to red cells surrounding the antibody-producing B cells. After addition of complement, these red cells lyse to leave a clear zone (plaque) around each specific B cell.

Elispot assays are conceptually similar to PFC assays but use ELISA-type detection systems. They can be used to enumerate antibody-producing B cells, by culturing them on plates sensitized with specific antigen. Antibody binds to the plate in a spot around the secreting B cell and the spots are visualized by developing the plate with enzyme conjugated anti-immunoglobulin and chromogen. Alternatively the method can be used for detecting cytokine-producing T cells. The plate is sensitized with one cytokine-specific antibody, which captures the secreted cytokine. This is then detected with another cytokine-specific antibody in a manner analogous to capture immunoassays.

Chemotaxis assays are occasionally used to assess macrophage or polymorph function. The cells are placed on one side of a millipore filter, and chemotactic agents on the other (e.g. C5a, LTB4, f-Met. Leu. PhE tripeptide). Numbers of migrating cells are usually assessed microscopically.

Candida-**killing assay** is used to assess the ability of macrophages to kill endocytosed organisms.

Neutrophil function assays are generally designed to detect the respiratory burst which normally occurs after endocytosis of opsonized material. Most widely used is the nitroblue tetrazolium (NBT) reduction assay in which normal neutrophils generate a blue endproduct. During the respiratory burst chemiluminescence is also detectable, and oxygen radical generation occurs. The ability of neutrophils to kill endocytosed organisms may be detected by culture with *Staphylococcus aureus,* and enumerating surviving bacteria.

Complement assays The simplest measure of complement activity is the CH50 test which measures the highest dilution of serum which will lyse 50% of antibody-sensitized erythrocytes. This is relatively crude, as it depends on the combined action of many complement components. It is possible to modify the CH50 assay to estimate the functional activity of individual complement components, in similar assays. However, this requires specialist reagents, so individual components are more usually measured by radioimmunoassay or ELISA.

Appendix 1:
Immunoglobulin levels

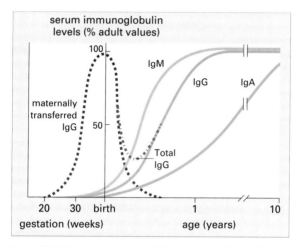

Appendix 1.1 Serum immunoglobulin levels and age. Maternally transferred IgG has mostly disappeared by 6 months. As the neonate actively synthesizes IgG the level slowly rises, but a physiological 'trough' of serum IgG is characteristically seen between 3 and 6 months.

Appendix 2:
Principal CD markers and principal cytokines

Principal CD markers		
CD	*Identity/function*	*Main cell types expressing:*
CD1	Unknown	Cortical thymocytes
CD2	LFA-3 receptor	Mature T cells
CD3	T cell receptor	Mature T cells
CD4	MHC class II receptor	T cell subset
CD5	CD72 receptor	T cells; B cell subset
CD8	MHC class I receptor	T cell subset
CD11a	LFA-1 (α chain)	All leucocytes
CD11b	CR3 = Mac1 (α chain)	Monocyte/macrophage neutrophil
CD14	LPS receptor	Monocyte/macrophage
CD15	binds ELAM-1	Macrophage; granulocyte
CD16	Fcγ receptor (type III)	Phagocytes; platelets; LGLs
CD18	LFA-1 and CR3 (β chain)	All leucocytes
CD21	CR2 complement receptor	B cell subset
CD23	Fcε receptor (low aff.)	B cell subset
CD25	IL-2 receptor	Activated T or B cell
CD29	VLA-integrins (β chain)	All leucocytes
CD32	Fcγ receptor (type II)	B cell; mononuclear phagocytes
CD35	CR1 complement receptor	B cell; mononuclear phagocytes
CD45	Leucocyte common antigen	All leucocytes
CD45R	Restricted LCA	T cell subsets; other leucocytes
CD46	MCP	All leucocytes
CD49a–f	VLA-integrins (α chains)	Variable
CD54	ICAM-1	Activated leucocytes
CD55	DAF	All leucocytes
CD56	NCAM	LGLs; activated lymphocytes
CD58	LFA-3 (CD2 receptor)	All leucocytes
CD64	Fcγ receptor (type I)	Mononuclear phagocytes
CD71	Transferrin receptor	Activated lymphocyte; macrophage
CD72	CD5 receptor	B cells

CR: complement receptor; DAF: decay accelerating factor; ELAM-1: endothelial leucocyte adhesion molecule; ICAM: intercellular adhesion molecule; LFA: lymphocyte functional antigen; LPS: lipopolysaccharide; MCP: membrane cofactor protein; NCAM: neural cell adhesion molecule; VLA: very late antigen.

Principal cytokines			
Cytokines	Sources	Targets	Main effects
IL-1α	Macrophages Lymphocytes	Lymphocytes Macrophages	Pro-inflammatory Cytokine production; endothelial activation
IL-1β	Epithelia Astrocytes	Fibroblasts Endothelium	Cytokine receptor induction Phagocyte activation
IL-2	T cells	T cells B cells	Required for division
IL-4 IL-5	T cells	B cells	Required for division and differentiation
IL-6	Macrophages Fibroblasts	T cells B cells	Promote differentiation
	T cells Endothelium	Hepatocytes Other cells	Acute phase proteins Pro-inflammatory
IL-10	T cell subset	T cell subset	Blocks cytokine production
IFN-γ	T cells	Macrophages Other cells Endothelium	Activation MHC induction Activation
TNF-α	Macrophages Lymphocytes	Lymphocytes Monocytes	Activation
TNF-β	T cells	NK cells Endothelium	Enhances cytotoxicity Activation; pro-inflammatory
TGF-β	T cells B cells	T cells B cells	Inhibits activation

Appendix 3:
Vaccination schedules

Vaccine	Age	Notes
Diphtheria (D/T/P) Tetanus Pertussis Haemophilus infl type B	2 months 3 months 4 months	primary course
Measles/mumps/ rubella	12–18 months	give at any age over 12 months
Booster D/T and polio MMR (if not already given)	4–5 years	
Rubella	10–14 years	GIRLS ONLY
BCG	10–14 years or infancy	leave 3 weeks between BCG & rubella
Booster tetanus and polio	15–18 years	

Children should have received the following vaccines

By 6 months	3 doses of D/T/P, Hib and polio
By 15 months	measles/mumps/rubella
By school entry	4th D/T and polio; measles/mumps/rubella if not already given
Between 10 and 14 years	BCG; and rubella for girls
Before leaving school	5th polio and tetanus

Adults should receive the following vaccines

Women seronegative for rubella	rubella
Unimmunized individuals	polio, tetanus
Individuals in high risk groups	hepatitis B, hepatitis A, influenza

ANAPHYLAXIS

Anaphylactic reactions are seen following immunization and patients should be kept under observation to make sure no reaction occurs.

Measles/mumps/rubella
Special care should be taken with this vaccine and it should not be given to children with proven allergy to egg who have experienced anaphylactic to that food. Dislike is not a contraindication. It should not be given if there is an allergy to neomycin or kanamycin.

Derived from *Immunisation against Infectious Disease* (1992) HMSO, London.

Appendix: 4
HLA haplotypes
and frequencies

Allele	European caucasoids (228)	African blacks (102)	Japanese (195)
B5	5.9	3.0	20.9
B7	10.4	7.3	7.1
B8	9.2	7.1	0.2
B12	16.6	12.7	6.5
B13	3.2	1.5	0.8
B14	2.4	3.6	0.5
B18	6.2	2.0	—
B27	4.6	—	0.3
B15	4.8	3.0	9.3
Bw38 ⎤ Bw16	2.0	—	1.8
Bw39 ⎦	3.5	1.5	4.7
B17	5.7	16.1	0.6
Bw21	2.2	1.5	1.5
Bw22	3.6	—	6.5
Bw35	9.9	7.2	9.4
B37	1.1	—	0.8
B40	8.1	2.0	21.8
Bw41	1.2	1.5	—
Bw42	—	12.3	—
blank	2.4	17.9	7.6

Appendix 4.1 HLA-B locus gene frequencies (%). Population differences in HLA haplotypes.